Praise For Dr. Now Book

~~~~~~~~This Isn't A Diet, It Is So Much More!~~~~~~`

"What I love about this book is that it brings healthy ingredients to the forefront, without being snobby. The section on now diet-friendly alternatives is particularly useful, and every recipe is just 6 carbs! That's some no-brainer type of now diet stuff I can get behind."—Amanda C. Hughes

Awesome information

"This book was incredibly helpful for a dr now diet newbie. I love that there are shopping lists that coordinate with the recipes!"—Nancy T.

Delicious recipes, healthy eating!!

"The author was informative and had a strong knowledge on Dr. Now Diet. I feel like this book has equipped me to be knowledgeable and successful with my new Now Diet low carb journey. Highly recommend this book to others."—Ccoard

Excellent book with wonderful recipes

"I enjoy this book because it discusses a concise, well-researched diet that uses foods I already buy on a weekly basis and focuses more on natural foods such as fruits, nuts, and veggies. This diet plan is already helping me reach my goal."—Meistjac

Must have book for a better life

"This book is very practical. It provides tips to slowly include changes to create sustainable habits, not only in eating, but in exercise, and other relaxing lifestyle behaviors. My husband even made the comment that this could be an eating plan he could stick to, enjoy and lose weight."—Wanda S

Dr. Nowzaradan Diet Plan Book For Beginners.

28 Days Meal Plan And 1000 Affordable Recipes for Healthy Living

Catharine Smith

Disclaimer

Dedication

*We dedicate this book to the complete
Catharine Smith team,
Supporters, well-wishers and
The Catharine Smith community.*

*It goes without saying that we
would not have gotten
this far without
encouragement,
critique and support*

Table Of Contents

Cause Of Obesity And It's Solution

If you want to lose weight, the general advice you are given is to eat less and move more. It seems very simple but why doesn't it work? We need to understand the disease of obesity from the beginning. Let's understand obesity the same way we understand any disease. We must understand what causes obesity. We have focused more on the answer than on the cause. But now let us understand the reason. One of the causes of obesity is that obesity is often genetic. Obesity in your family determines 70% of your chances of gaining weight. However, only 30% of the factors we can influence are in our hands. What should we do now? Is diet and exercise the only answer?

We are obsessed with how many calories we consume. But we don't think much about how many calories we burn. Because it is a bit difficult to measure how many calories we expend. The total energy expenditure is the sum of basal metabolic rates, thermogenic effects of food, non-exercise thermogenesis, post-exercise excess oxygen consumption, and exercise.

We believe that all calories are equal. But no two foods have the same response after entering the body. There can be clearly distinguishable differences between the two substances. For example sugar and olive oil. Sugar will raise blood glucose and trigger an insulin response from your pancreas. Olive oil will not. There is no increase in blood sugar or insulin after olive oil is absorbed through the small intestine. Both foods trigger vastly different hormonal reactions and metabolic responses.

All the food we eat contains calories. When food is first ingested in the stomach, it is mixed with stomach acid and slowly released into the small intestine. Nutrients are removed from both small and large intestines and Rest is excreted as stool. Carbohydrates are broken down directly into their building blocks sugars.

Imagine that you consume 2100 calories of energy in a day. How can these 2100 calories be metabolized? These calories can be used for many purposes.

- Heat production
- new protein production,
- New bone production
- new muscle production,
- cognition (brain),
- Increased heart rate
- Increased stroke volume (heart),
- exercise/physical exertion,
- Detoxification (liver)
- detoxification (kidney),
- Digestive system (pancreas & bowels).
- breathing (lungs),
- excretion (intestines & colon)
- Fat production

We are not happy when our body stores calories as fat. We think that fat gain is arbitrary and weight loss is governed by the calorie-balance system model. But this is not the case for every system in your body. Hormones regulate every system in the body. Many systems are at work to control your body weight.

Fat storage is a form of calorie distribution. The production of fat consumes a lot of calories. This energy expenditure can be controlled almost completely automatically. You can't count how many calories it takes to gain fat. There are two key responses to losing weight. In order to preserve energy, the total energy expenditure must be immediately and indefinitely decreased.

Hormonal hunger signals are immediately amplified. Losing weight makes us hungry and slows down our metabolism. It is your natural physical activity that will help you gain the lost weight. It has nothing to do with our lack of willpower. It is part of the normal hormones in our body. We eat more because our brain tells our body to eat more.

We do what our hormones tell us to do. However, our friends, family, medical professionals and others silently blame the victim believing that it is "our fault." We also feel that we are failures. Are you familiar with this? All dieters have the same sad story of losing or regaining weight. The science behind the cycle is well established and millions of dieters have seen its truth. However, nutrition experts believe that calorie reduction leads to permanent weight loss.

Until now we believed that exercise is very important for weight loss. That is, we believed that if we increased our exercise, we would burn more calories. Traditional diet and exercise are two methods that are recommended for weight loss. Also, neither exercise nor diet are fifty-fifty partners in weight loss.

Diet is 95% important so we need to pay all attention to diet. Exercise is good, it has many benefits, but weight loss is not. Don't expect yourself to lose weight by exercising. If you focus all your research, money, time, mental energy on exercise, you will not be able to fight obesity. Excess calories do not cause obesity, hormonal imbalances cause obesity. Hormones regulate many body systems and processes, including appetite, fat storage, and blood levels.

The hormone leptin is not responsible for controlling your body weight. One of the reasons why we become fat is that we increase our food intake. Health professionals now encourage snacking, but in the past, snacking was strongly discouraged. Snacking is a great way to eat, according to researchers. But since we eat sugary snacks and high calorie snacks, we don't lose weight even by snacking. After all, my grandmother was right as she always said that snacking can make us fat. Because we often eat processed snacks that deprive our body of nutrients.

At breakfast time, ask your mind if you are hungry. And if the answer is no, then stop eating breakfast. If you are not hungry after eating a small amount of food in the morning, you should avoid eating too much in the morning. Also we should avoid eating refined carbohydrates and sugary foods. If we want to lose weight, we must not only eat a healthy diet, we must also replace the less healthy foods we eat with a healthy diet.

As our tendency to eat more has increased the rate of obesity. Also obesity is a hormonal disorder that regulates fat. Insulin is the main hormone responsible for weight gain. The solution is to lower insulin levels. To do this, lower insulin levels by using all the options available to you. First we need to remove sugar from our dining room. You don't need to add sugar to any food or drink.

Some processed foods contain almost 100% sugar. Some people eat sugar on their own. That's why we should focus our efforts on reducing added sugars instead of natural sugars. Two major findings have emerged from the periodic weight loss diet research. The first is that every diet works. The second is that all diets fail. What does this mean?

Permanent weight loss is an ongoing process. This is a short-term and long-term problem. The part of the brain responsible for determining the set weight of the body. Insulin determines upper body weight. The short-term problem is losing weight and the long-term problem is not regaining the lost weight.

Science Behind The Dr Now Diet

All animals and most species can't choose their food as human beings. Because they don't have the freedom to choose food by variety, type, and quantity. In simple words, cows and buffaloes are attracted to grass as of their inbuilt food instinct. But human beings don't have one fixed food instinct, we can choose our food based on our judgment and this is opposite to the theory of evolution.

Every culture and society worldwide has different food choices that are majorly different. So it is impossible to have one diet with the same suitable recipes worldwide. The food intake and dietary balance in animals are stronger than in human beings, preventing them from overeating. So animals eat only to survive! When we are newborns through infancy, we have an efficient regulatory mechanism of food intake that prevents us from overeating, but as we get older, our regulatory mechanism becomes inactive.

Today's dietary lifestyle has reduced the amount of vitamins and minerals in our bodies. Fewer vitamins are needed for our daily activities. Many diets have been popular for centuries. Each diet becomes popular only for 2-3 years. First we need to understand why every diet expires after 2-3 years and then we need a new diet.

When we start following a diet but we don't see the results immediately and even if we do, we can't stick to the results. As a result, we go back to our old habits and gain weight. Another reason is that every diet comes with a list of suggested foods that usually don't match the list of foods you eat. We follow a diet, but it gets boring, and when it gets boring, we go back to our old habits, and the cravings come back, and the weight we lost is put back on. For long-term weight loss, we must adopt healthy eating habits. Healthy eating habits require timely, regular meals. We should practice chewing food 32 times.

Follow the 20-minute rule for each meal, and don't watch TV and computer at mealtime. We must avoid fast food and food eating due to stress and boredom. Don't eat snacks in between two meals. Drink one glass of water before each meal, this will make us feel full earlier, and we will eat less. Ultimately our calorie intake lowers. We need to pay attention to the nutritional labeling of packaged foods. Remind yourself of the serving size. Usually, the purpose of serving sizes is to provide you an appropriate amount of food to consume and not exceed more than one serving size.

Calories: calorie content is given per one serving size. For instance, if the calorie content of the nutrition label is 160 calories per serving size and there are 8 serving sizes per package, then the content is equal to 1280 calories.

What Is Dr Now Diet

Dr now introduces a new rule to our eating habits.

There are three aspects that affect our daily intake of calories. These three factors are what dr now refers it as the acronym F.A.T.

F stands for frequency, A stands for amount, and T stands for the type of food.

Frequency- The frequency of eating habits should be 2 or 3 meals a day. Do not have snacks in between meals.

Amount- The amount limits our calorie intake per day to 1200 calories, and each meal should have about 400 calories per day.

Type- meal should be nutritious and protein-rich as well as low in calories and carbs and high in fiber.

Developing own dr now diet plan

The best diet for us is what we develop for ourselves. We have created steps to create your own dr now diet plan. First, make a list of your favorite foods for breakfast, lunch, and dinner. Second, remove all high-calorie foods from the list.

High-calorie foods to avoid:

Sugar, Chocolate, Crackers, Potato chips, Potatoes, French fries, Mashed Potatoes, and tater tots, Popcorn, Peanut butter, almonds, cashews, Pistachios, Sunflower seeds

Candy, cookies, cake, donuts, pies, ice cream, sweetened fruit, and frozen yogurt. Sherbet/sorbet, milkshakes, chocolate milk, pudding, and sweetened gelatin desserts
White rice and brown rice, Pasta and noodles, cereals

Fruit juices like orange juice, apple juice, cranberry juice, and grape juice.

Bread and tortillas, sodas or sugary drinks or energy drinks

Fruits like watermelon, cantaloupes, and bananas.

Honey syrup, molasses, and meal supplements have excessive carbohydrates and sugar in them.

The third step is to choose, mix and match our favorite food with 400 calories per meal.

4 ounces of grilled chicken breast has 187 calories.
4 ounces of tuna have 209 calories.
One cup of tomato soup has 72 calories.
One boiled egg has 78 calories.
One cup of fat-free yogurt has 95 calories.
So, with very little effort and some homework, we can create our favorite diet plan that is nutritional, satisfying, and sustainable. So far, our own diet is the best diet.

Dr Now Diet Shopping Guide

Clean Out Your Pantry

According to researchers, if there are unhealthy foods in our home, we are more likely to eat those foods and we tend to eat them. If you don't live alone, be sure to talk about your housemates and be aware of them. Be it your significant other or family member or roommate. And some foods that are unhealthy but you can't take them out of the house. So at least keep it out of your sight in another room. Make sure you keep unhealthy foods out of the house to show you're committed to starting your new diet.

STARCHES AND GRAINS

Eliminate everything: pasta, cereal rice, potatoes, corn, oats, quinoa bread, bagels, flour wraps, rolls, and croissants.

SUGARY FOODS AND DRINKS

Eliminate any refined sugar and fruit juices, fountain drinks and milk pastries, desserts, and chocolates made from milk and candy bars.

LEGUMES

Eliminate beans, peas, and lentils. They're loaded with carbs. One cup of beans contains greater than 3 times more carbohydrates than you should consume every day.

PROCESSED POLYUNSATURATED FATS AND OILS

Eliminate most seed oils such as any soybean, safflower, vegetable, sunflower, and corn oils. Eliminate trans fats, such as anything hydrogenated or partially hydrogenated.

FRUITS

Eliminate any fruits high in carbohydrates such as mangoes, grapes, dates, bananas, apples and mangoes. Get rid of raisins. Avoid eating dried fruits as they contain the same amount of sugar as regular fruits. But they are more concentrated. For example, one cup of grapefruit contains 20 grams of carbohydrates. One cup of raisins contains more than 100 grams of carbohydrates.

Go Shopping

It's time to stock up your refrigerator, pantry, and freezer with Doctor Nowzaradan's delicious treats. Which will help you experience weight loss and improve your health.

THE BASICS

If you have these basic ingredients in your kitchen with these essentials, you'll always be able to cook delicious, healthy dishes and snacks.

Coffee, water, and tea
The spices, herbs, and all the other ingredients
Sweeteners, such as stevia and the erythritol
Lime juice or lemon juice

Low-carb condiments such as mayonnaise, pesto, mustard, and Sriracha
Broths (chicken bones, beef)
Fermented and pickled foods such as pickles, kimchi, and sauerkraut
Nuts and seeds include macadamia nuts and pecans, hazelnuts, walnuts and almonds, flaxseed, pine nuts, Chia seeds, and pumpkin seeds.

MEATS

All types of meat are suitable for Dr. Nowzaradan's diet. In which all types of meat like chicken, pork, beef, lamb, turkey are better if they come in the budget. You can take and eat the fat from chicken skin and meat. Wild seafood and fish are fine just avoid farmed fish. Have fun with eggs.

VEGGIES

You can eat all vegetables like asparagus, mushroom, broccoli, cucumber, onion, pepper, tomato, garlic. Because there is no starch in it. Avoid starchy foods like yams, potatoes.

Guide To Eating Outside On Dr Now Diet

Brunch: Traditional brunch dishes include scrambled eggs, bacon, sausage, steak and eggs, and omelets. Also avoid fruit juice as much as possible. Because it is high in sugar. You can continue drinking unsweetened tea and water or coffee.

Lunch at work : Bringing your own lunch to work can be a great option to help you live a healthy lifestyle together. We should take a lunch break with colleagues. Try to keep these tips in mind.

Read the menu before going out to eat. By preparing ahead of time, eating out reduces the amount of stress that comes with it. Also remember that you should consume 400 calories per meal.

Include more protein in your meals. Also, include healthy fats and vegetables in your meals that are nutritious for your body. Salads are great -- ask for no croutons and opt for olive oil and vinegar instead of a sugar-laden salad dressing

Be sure to keep grains and starches off your table to avoid temptation. When you order an entree, replace them with vegetables or salads that you steam.

It is difficult not to join the BBQ gathering but by following some dietary rules we can join and enjoy the BBQ gathering. Options that are approved by Dr. Now includes brisket, sausage, barbecued fish, smoked chicken, and ribs, as well as grilled low-carb fruits and vegetables. Also, consider sugar-free sauces and seasonings instead of the teriyaki sauce as well as BBQ sauce.

Buffet: The buffet method is my favorite because the buffet method provides you with a variety of healthy menu items. Think grilling seafood, steamed vegetables, chicken. Be sure to avoid starchy vegetables like beans, potatoes, and parsnips. Also avoid sugary salad dressings.

Do you dread eating out whenever there's a holiday party? If the answer is yes, then there is no reason to panic if you follow a diet plan approved by a nutritionist.

Do not leave your stomach empty before going out to eat. Eat some food. By doing this we can avoid breadbaskets and sugary foods. Don't be afraid to say no. If you don't want to eat a food and are being pressured to eat it, don't be shy about saying no.

Don't forget to go out to eat and have fun. Enjoy the meal. Enjoy the people you are with without stressing yourself out. Remember that even if you don't eat 100% of Dr. nowzaradan's food, you can get back on track with the next meal.

28 Days Meal Plan

WEEK 1 MEAL PLAN

MONDAY

Breakfast: Almond Cereal – Page No. 3

Lunch: Feta & Sun-Dried Tomato Salad - Page No. 53

Dinner: Chicken "Ramen" Soup - Page No. 54

Per Day Calories: 1002; Fat: 88; Protein: 59g; Net Carbs: 19g

TUESDAY

Breakfast: Mushroom Omelet- Page No. 5

Lunch: Pesto Caprese Salad with Tuna - Page No. 55

Dinner: Chicken Noodle Soup - Page No. 55

Per Day Calories: 1108; Fat: 76g; Protein: 68g; Net Carbs: 16g

WEDNESDAY

Breakfast: Creamy Eggs and Asparagus - Page No. 2

Lunch: Salmon Stew- Page No. 56

Dinner: Spicy Halibut Tomato Soup - Page No. 58

Per Day Calories: 1008; Fat: 72g; Protein: 77g; Net Carbs: 22g

THURSDAY

Breakfast: Chili Tomatoes and Eggs - Page No. 2

Lunch: Spinach & Brussels Sprout Salad - Page No. 57

Dinner: Cheesy Zucchini Soup- Page No. 60

Per Day Calories: 1148; Fat: 69g; Protein: 79g; Net Carbs: 20g

FRIDAY

Breakfast: Breakfast Bowl - Page No. 6

Lunch: Rosemary Chicken with Avocado Sauce - Page No.

Dinner: Rosemary Beef Meatza - Page No. 209

Per Day Calories: 978; Fat: 78g; Protein: 85g; Net Carbs: 14g

SATURDAY

Breakfast: Zesty Zucchini Bread with Nuts - Page No. 7

Lunch: Chorizo in Cabbage Sauce with Pine Nuts - Page No. 151

Dinner: Pork Soup - Page No. 191

Per Day Calories: 1033; Fat: 67g; Protein: 81g; Net Carbs: 14g

SUNDAY

Breakfast: Eggs and Sausages - Page No. 9

Lunch: Bell Pepper & Beef Sausage Frittata- Page No. 194

Dinner: Chicken Pasta - Page No. 148

Per Day Calories: 1056; Fat: 76g; Protein: 79g; Net Carbs: 14g

WEEK 2 MEAL PLAN

MONDAY

Breakfast: Ham & Cheese Sandwiches - Page No. 9

Lunch: Creamy Leek & Salmon Soup - Page No. 58

Dinner: Cabbage Soup - Page No. 61

Per Day Calories: 1040; Fat: 72g; Protein: 79g; Net Carbs: 15g

TUESDAY

Breakfast: Spinach and Eggs Salad - Page No. 10

Lunch: Thai Coconut Soup with Shrimp- Page No. 59

Dinner: Mint Avocado Chilled Soup - Page No. 62

Per Day Calories: 975; Fat: 79g; Protein: 87g; Net Carbs: 16g

WEDNESDAY

Breakfast: Breakfast Muffins - Page No. 11

Lunch: Turkey Bacon & Turnip Salad - Page No. 60

Dinner: Thai Beef and Broccoli Soup - Page No. 63

Per Day Calories: 1007; Fat: 73g; Protein: 77g; Net Carbs: 17g

THURSDAY

Breakfast: Scrambled Eggs - Page No. 11

Lunch: Fiery Shrimp Cocktail Salad - Page No. 61

Dinner: Bacon Cheeseburger Soup - Page No. 64

Per Day Calories: 1037; Fat: 77g; Protein: 79g; Net Carbs: 20g

FRIDAY

Breakfast: Creamy Eggs - Page No. 13

Lunch: Chicken, Avocado & Egg Bowls - Page No. 62

Dinner: Taco Soup - Page No. 71

Per Day Calories: 1035; Fat: 74g; Protein: 85g; Net Carbs: 14g

SATURDAY

Breakfast: French Toast with Berry Yogurt - Page No. 15

Lunch: Seared Rump Steak Salad - Page No. 67

Dinner: Maple Jalapeño Beef Plate - Page No. 207

Per Day Calories: 1133; Fat: 77g; Protein: 81g; Net Carbs: 14g

SUNDAY

Breakfast: Chicken Breakfast Muffins - Page No. 17

Lunch: Cheesy Beef Salad - Page No. 68

Dinner: Sage Beef Meatloaf with Pecans - Page No. 205

Per Day Calories: 1112; Fat: 73g; Protein: 79g; Net Carbs: 14g

WEEK 3 MEAL PLAN

MONDAY

Breakfast: Breakfast Pork Bagel - Page No. 18

Lunch: Mediterranean Artichoke Salad - Page No. 63

Dinner: Five-Minute Creamy Tomato Soup - Page No. 74

Per Day Calories: 1140; Fat: 72g; Protein: 79g; Net Carbs: 25g

TUESDAY

Breakfast: Spinach Nests with Eggs & Cheese - Page No. 19

Lunch: Arugula & Watercress Turkey - Page No. 64

Dinner: Creamy Artichoke Soup - Page No. 76

Per Day Calories: 1125; Fat: 79g; Protein: 72g; Net Carbs: 16g

WEDNESDAY

Breakfast: Bacon & Mushroom "Tacos" - Page No. 20

Lunch: Spinach Salad with Goat Cheese & Nuts - Page No. 65

Dinner: Spiced Pumpkin Soup - Page No. 78

Per Day Calories: 1107; Fat: 73g; Protein: 77g; Net Carbs: 17g

THURSDAY

Breakfast: Tomato and Eggs Salad - Page No. 21

Lunch: Thai-Style Prawn Salad - Page No. 66

Dinner: Chicken Enchilada Soup - Page No. 79

Per Day Calories: 1137; Fat: 77g; Protein: 79g; Net Carbs: 20g

FRIDAY

Breakfast: Avocado Muffins - Page No. 22

Lunch: Seared Rump Steak Salad - Page No. 67

Dinner: Sausage-Pepper Soup - Page No. 80

Per Day Calories: 1135; Fat: 74g; Protein: 80g; Net Carbs: 14g

SATURDAY

Breakfast: Tuna & Egg Salad with Chili Mayo - Page No. 23

Lunch: Vietnamese Salad - Page No. 186

Dinner: Beef Taco - Page No. 200

Per Day Calories: 1133; Fat: 77g; Protein: 81g; Net Carbs: 14g

SUNDAY

Breakfast: Microwave Bacon Frittata - Page No. 24

Lunch: Delicious Pork Tenderloin - Page No. 184

Dinner: Gingery Pork Stir-Fry- Page No. 192

Per Day Calories: 1112; Fat: 74g; Protein: 79g; Net Carbs: 14g

WEEK 4 MEAL PLAN

MONDAY

Breakfast: Goat Cheese Frittata with Asparagus   - Page No. 27

Lunch: Taco Salad- Page No. 67

Dinner: Sausage And Pepper Soup - Page No. 82

Per Day Calories: 1140; Fat: 72g; Protein: 79g; Net Carbs: 25g

TUESDAY

Breakfast: Beef, Avocado and Eggs - Page No. 28

Lunch: Avocado and Chicken Salad - Page No. 68

Dinner: Chinese Tofu Soup - Page No. 83

Per Day Calories: 1125; Fat: 79g; Protein: 76g; Net Carbs: 16g

WEDNESDAY

Breakfast: Pork and Avocado Mix - Page No. 29

Lunch: Egg Salad with Avocado - Page No. 69

Dinner: Fresh Avocado-Cucumber Soup - Page No. 84

Per Day Calories: 1107; Fat: 33g; Protein: 77g; Net Carbs: 17g

THURSDAY

Breakfast: Pork and Avocado Mix - Page No. 30

Lunch: Cauliflower Salad - Page No. 69

Dinner: Easy Green Baby Spinach Soup - Page No. 85

Per Day Calories: 1137; Fat: 73g; Protein: 79g; Net Carbs: 20g

FRIDAY

Breakfast: Morning Herbed Eggs - Page No. 31

Lunch: Spinach and Watercress Salad- Page No. 70

Dinner: Awesome Zucchini Boats Stuffed with Beef- Page No. 204

Per Day Calories: 1135; Fat: 74g; Protein: 85g; Net Carbs: 14g

SATURDAY

Breakfast: Chili Spinach and Beef Mix - Page No. 34

Lunch: Swiss Pork Patties with Salad - Page No. 181

Dinner: Pork & Pumpkin Stew with Peanuts- Page No. 132

Per Day Calories: 1133; Fat: 77g; Protein: 81g; Net Carbs: 14g

SUNDAY

Breakfast: Spinach Omelet- Page No. 38

Lunch: Zucchini & Bell Pepper Chicken Gratin - Page No. 141

Dinner: Crusted Pork Loin- Page No. 182

Per Day Calories: 998; Fat: 73g; Protein: 79g; Net Carbs: 14g

Breakfast

Creamy Eggs and Asparagus

Preparation time: 10 minutes

Cooking time: 15 minutes

Servings: 4

Ingredients:

- 2 ounces butter
- 4 eggs, whisked
- 8 ounces coconut cream
- 3 ounces parmesan, grated
- A pinch of salt and black pepper
- A pinch of cayenne pepper
- 1 and ½ pounds green asparagus, trimmed and halved
- 1 and ½ tablespoon lemon juice
- 1 tablespoon olive oil

Directions:

In a pan, melt butter over medium-high temperature, add the eggs and mix them for about 6 to 7 minutes. Add cream, parmesan, salt, pepper, and cayenne, mix until well, then take off the heat and divide between plates. In a pan, heat the oil at medium-high and add asparagus as well as one pinch of cayenne, and lemon juice. Cook for about 2 minutes each side. Then divide it among scrambled eggs and serve for breakfast. Enjoy!

Nutrition: calories 212, fat 8, fiber 5, carbs 15, protein 7

Crespelle al Mascarpone

Ingredients for 2 servings

- ½ cup almond flour
- 2 tsp liquid stevia
- 1 tsp baking powder
- ½ cup almond milk
- 1 tsp vanilla extract
- 1 large egg
- ¼ cup olive oil
- Whole raspberries to garnish
- 1 cup mascarpone cheese
- 1 tsp mint, chopped

Directions and Total Time: approx. 35 minutes

Mix the eggs in an egg bowl. Add the vanilla extract, almond milk along with half of the stevia. mix to combine. In a different bowl, whisk both baking and almond flour together. Then, add an egg mix into the mixture of almond flour, and continue to whisk until it is smooth. Place olive oil in the pan on moderate heat. Pour into 1 soup spoon of batter. Cook one side for two minutes, flip the pancake and cook the second side for two minutes. Transfer the pancake onto an oven-safe plate, and repeat the cooking procedure until the batter is totally absorbed. Mix the mascarpone and the remaining mint and stevia in a small bowl. Make every mini pancake in mascarpone. Then sprinkle the raspberry over for serving.

Per serving: Cal 717; Net Carbs 6.2g; Fat 61g; Protein 35g

Chili Tomatoes and Eggs

Ingredients for 4 servings:

- 4 eggs, whisked   2 shallots, chopped
- 4 tomatoes, cubed   2 chili peppers, minced
- 1 tablespoon ghee, melted
- Salt and black pepper to the taste
- 1 teaspoon sweet paprika
- 1 tablespoon chives, chopped

Instructions (10 min preparation time, 20 min cooking time):

Prepare a pan using the ghee at medium-high temperature, add the shallots and the chili peppers, mix and cook for 5 mins. Add the tomatoes and all the other ingredients, excluding eggs, mix well and cook the mixture for another 5 minutes. Include the egg, stir little bit and cook for 5 more minutes, then divide the mix between plates before serving.

Nutrition: calories 119, fat 7.9, fiber 1.8, carbs 6.5, protein 6.9

Jalapeño Waffles with Bacon & Avocado

Ingredients for 4 servings

- 2 tbsp butter, melted
- ¼ cup almond milk
- 2 tbsp almond flour
- Salt and black pepper to taste
- ½ tsp parsley, chopped
- ½ jalapeño pepper, minced
- 4 eggs ½ cup cheddar, crumbled
- 4 slices bacon, chopped
- 1 avocado, sliced

Directions and Total Time: approx. 20 minutes

In a pan over medium-high heat, fry the bacon until crisp for approximately 5 minutes. Transfer onto the plate. Put in a bowl mix all the ingredients except for avocado. Heat the waffle iron, and spray it using cooking spray. Pour the batter into the iron and seal the lid. Bake for about 5 mins. Repeat the process with the remaining batter. Add bacon and avocado.

Per serving: Cal 641; Net Carbs 6g; Fat 58g; Protein 24g 35.

Almond Cereal

Preparation time: 5 minutes

Cooking time: 0 minutes.

Servings: 2

Ingredients:

- 2 tablespoons almonds, chopped
- 2 tablespoons sunflower seeds, roasted
- ⅓ cup coconut milk
- 1 tablespoon chia seeds
- ⅓ cup water
- ½ cup blueberries

Directions:

In a bowl, mix the chia seeds and coconut milk and then set aside for five minutes. In a food processor, blend one tablespoon of sunflower seeds and almonds and process them thoroughly. Add this mixture to the chia seeds mixture. Add water then stir. Top with the rest of the blueberries, sunflower seeds and serve.

Nutritional Value: Calories – 181, Fat – 15.2, Fiber – 4, Carbs – 10.8, Protein – 3.7

Perfect Buttermilk Pancakes

Ingredients for 4 servings

- 3 eggs
- 1 cup buttermilk
- 1 cup almond flour
- ½ tsp baking powder
- 1 tbsp Swerve
- 1 lemon, juiced
- 1 vanilla pod
- 2 tbsp unsalted butter
- 3 tbsp sugar-free maple syrup

Directions and Total Time: approx. 25 minutes

In a small bowl, mix the buttermilk, lemon juice and eggs. In a separate bowl blend almond flour with baking powder and make sure to whisk. Add the egg mixture, and whisk until it is smooth. Slice the vanilla pod open and then scrape beans in the mix of flour. Stir until the mixture is well-integrated. Let the batter rest over 10 mins. Make a small amount of butter melt in a skillet on medium-low temperature. Pour about 1/4 cup of batter to each pancake. Cook for about 2 minutes or until tiny bubbles start to form. Then flip and cook for two minutes, or till it is set and golden. Repeat cooking process until the rest of the batter is done. Serve the pancakes on plates then drizzle them with maple syrup, then serve with a generous portion of yogurt and raspberries should you wish.

Per serving: Cal 330; Net Carbs 4.3g; Fat 18g; Protein 4g

Poached Eggs

Preparation time: 10 minutes

Cooking time: 35 minutes

Servings: 4

Ingredients:

- 3 garlic cloves, peeled and minced
- 1 tablespoon butter
- 1 white onion, peeled and chopped
- 1 Serrano pepper, chopped
- Salt and ground black pepper, to taste
- 1 red bell pepper, seeded and chopped
- 3 tomatoes, cored and chopped
- 1 teaspoon paprika
- 1 teaspoon cumin
- ¼ teaspoon chili powder
- 1 tablespoon fresh cilantro, chopped
- 6 eggs

Directions:

In a pan, melt butter at medium-low heat. Add onion, stir and cook for 10 mins. Then add Serrano pepper, garlic, Stir, cook for one minute. Add red bell peppers, mix to cook, for about 10 minutes. In addition, add tomatoes chili powder, pepper, cumin and paprika. Stir to cook, for about 10 minutes. Crack eggs into the pan and sprinkle with salt and pepper. Cover pan to cook on low for six minutes. Sprinkle with cilantro and serve.

Nutrition: Calories – 180, Fat – 10,9, Fiber – 2,5, Carbs – 10,5, Protein – 11,7

Belgium Waffles with Cheese Spread

Ingredients for 2 servings

- ½ cup cream cheese, softened
- 1 lemon, zested and juiced
- 2 tbsp liquid stevia
- 2 tbsp olive oil
- ½ cup almond milk
- 3 eggs
- ½ cup almond flour

Directions and Total Time: approx. 25 minutes

Within a bowl mix the cream cheese and lemon zest, lemon juice and stevia. In another bowl, whisk the almond milk, olive oil and eggs. Mix in almond flour and mix until there are no lumps. Allow the batter to sit for 5 minutes before letting it get thicker. Spray a waffle iron with cooking spray. Pour a quarter cup of batter in the waffle iron per waffle, and cook for 5 minutes. Repeat with the rest of the batter. Cut the waffles in quarters, then apply the lemon spread on two waffles, snap, and serve.

Per serving: Cal 532; Net Carbs 11g; Fat 46g; Protein 18g

Breakfast Burger

Preparation time: 10 minutes
Cooking time: 15 minutes
Servings: 4

Ingredients:
- 1 pound beef, ground
- 1 teaspoon mustard
- ½ teaspoon onion powder
- ½ teaspoon garlic powder
- 2 tablespoons ghee
- A pinch of salt and black pepper
- ¼ cup homemade mayonnaise
- 1 teaspoon chili sauce

Directions:
In a bowl mix the meat with onions, mustard, garlic powder along with salt and pepper. Make four burgers from this mixture. Cook a pan using the ghee on medium-high heat adding the burgers, cook for about 4-5 minutes on each side, then divide them between plates and serve with mayonnaise spread and chili sauce over the top.

Nutrition: calories 200, fat 7, fiber 8, carbs 16, protein 29

Spinach & Feta Cheese Pancakes

Ingredients for 2 servings

- ½ cup almond flour
- ½ tsp baking powder
- ½ cup feta cheese, crumbled
- ½ cup spinach, chopped
- 2 tbsp coconut milk
- 1 egg, beaten

Directions and Total Time: approx. 20 minutes

Within a large bowl add the egg and almond flour, baking powder, coconut milk, and spinach. Whisk to mix. Place a skillet on moderate heat for about a minute. Grab a spoonful of soup of the mix then cook the mixture for two minutes. Flip the pancake and cook further for 1 minute. Remove onto a plate and repeat the cooking process until the batter is exhausted. Serve with your favorite topping.

Per serving: Cal 312; Net Carbs 4.3g; Fat 28g; Protein 14g

Mushroom Omelet

Ingredients for 4 servings:
- 2 spring onions, chopped
- ½ pound white mushrooms
- Salt and black pepper to the taste
- 4 eggs, whisked
- 1 tablespoon olive oil
- ½ teaspoon cumin, ground
- 1 tablespoon cilantro, chopped

Instructions: (10 minutes preparation time, 20 minutes cooking time):
Prepare a pan using the oil on medium temperature, add spring onions and mushrooms. Toss and cook for 5 mins. Add eggs, along with the other ingredients, mix gently and then pour onto the pan, then cover and cook on moderate heat for about 15 minutes. Cut the omelet into slices, divide it into plates, and serve it for

breakfast.

Nutrition: calories 109, fat 8.1, fiber 0.8, carbs 2.9, protein 7.5

Ginger Pancakes

Ingredients for 2 servings

- 1 cup almond flour
- 1 tsp cinnamon powder
- 2 tbsp Swerve
- ¼ tsp baking soda
- 1 tsp ginger powder
- 1 egg
- 1 cup almond milk
- 2 tbsp olive oil Lime sauce
- ¼ cup liquid stevia
- ½ tsp arrowroot starch
- ½ lime, juiced and zested
- 2 tbsp butter

Directions and Total Time: approx. 20 minutes

Mix all the cinnamon powder, almond flour, baking soda, Swerve, egg, ginger powder, almond milk along with olive oil into an mixing bowl. Heat oil in a skillet over medium heat and spoon 2-3 tablespoons of the mixture into the skillet. Make the pancake for about 1 minute, then flip it and cook the second side for a further minute. Transfer the pancake to a raw plate. Repeat making the pancake until it has been exhausted. Mix the arrowroot starch and stevia in a saucepan. Set the saucepan over moderate heat, and slowly stir in 1 cup of water until it has thickened around 1 minute. Switch off the heat then add lime juice, butter and lime zest. Mix the ingredients to melt the butter. Serve the sauce on top of the pancakes and serve warm.

Per serving: Cal 443; Net Carbs 11g; Fat 38g; Protein 8g

Nutty Breakfast Bowl

Preparation time: 5 minutes

Cooking time: 0 minutes

Servings: 1

Ingredients:

- 1 teaspoon pecans, chopped
- ½ cup coconut milk
- 1 teaspoon walnuts, chopped
- 1 teaspoon pistachios, chopped
- 1 teaspoon almonds, chopped

- 1 teaspoon pine nuts, raw
- 1 teaspoon sunflower seeds, raw
- 1 teaspoon stevia
- 2 teaspoons raspberries

Directions:

In a bowl, mix milk with honey and stir. Add walnuts, pecans, almonds, pistachios and almonds. Add pine sunflower seeds. Stir well, garnish with raspberries, then serve.

Nutritional Value: Calories – 435, Fat – 44.2, Fiber – 5.2, Carbs – 10.8, Protein – 6.2

Peanut Butter & Pastrami Gofres

Ingredients for 2 servings
- 4 eggs
- ½ tsp baking soda
- 2 tbsp peanut butter, melted
- 4 tbsp coconut flour
- ¼ tsp salt
- ½ tsp dried rosemary
- 3 tbsp tomato puree
- 4 oz pastrami, chopped

Directions and Total Time: approx. 20 minutes

Preheat your waffle maker to high. Mix in a bowl and thoroughly mix your eggs with rosemary and salt. Add the coconut flour, baking soda, the coconut flour along with peanut butter. Continue whisking until the ingredients are thoroughly mixed. Add one third of the batter to the waffle iron , and bake for three minutes or until the waffle iron is golden. Repeat with the rest of the batter. Serve.

Per serving: Cal 411; Net Carbs 8g; Fat 27g; Protein 25g

Breakfast Bowl

Preparation time: 10 minutes

Cooking time: 20 minutes

Servings: 1

Ingredients:

- 4 ounces ground beef
- 1 onion, peeled and chopped
- 8 mushrooms, sliced

- Salt and ground black pepper, to taste
- 2 eggs, whisked
- 1 tablespoon coconut oil
- ½ teaspoon smoked paprika
- 1 avocado, pitted, peeled, and chopped
- 12 black olives, pitted and sliced

Directions:

In a pan, heat coconut oil on medium-high heat. Add mushrooms, onions, salt and pepper. Stir, and cook for five minutes. Add the beef and paprika. Stir, and cook for 10 mins, then transfer into a bowl. Heat up the pan again over medium heat, add eggs, some salt, pepper, and scramble. Return the beef mixture to the pan and mix. Add olives and avocados, stir, then cook for one minute. Transfer the mixture to a bowl and serve.

Nutrition: Calories – 1002, Fat – 74,9, Fiber – 19,4, Carbs – 36,9, Protein – 55,6

Savory Waffles with Cheese & Tomato

Ingredients for 2 servings
- 2 eggs, beaten
- 2 tbsp sour cream
- ¼ tsp allspice
- Salt and black pepper to taste
- 1/3 cup Gouda cheese, grated 1 tomato, sliced

Directions and Total Time: approx. 20 minutes

Combine the eggs, spices, salt, black pepper and sour cream in a shallow bowl. Add in the shredded cheese. Spritz a waffle iron with a cooking spray. Pour in half of the batter. Cook in the oven for five minutes or until the batter is golden. Repeat with the rest of the batter. Then serve with slices of tomato.

Per serving: Cal 254; Net Carbs 3.7g; Fat 18g; Protein 17g

Breakfast Cauliflower Mix

Preparation time: 10 minutes

Cooking time: 25 minutes

Servings: 4

Ingredients:

- 2 tablespoons ghee

- 1 small yellow onion, chopped
- 2 garlic cloves, minced
- 3 jalapeno peppers, chopped
- 1 pound beef meat, lean and ground
- A pinch of salt and black pepper
- 1 cauliflower head, grated
- ½ cup water
- ½ cup homemade mayonnaise
- ¼ cup sunflower seed butter
- 1 teaspoon cumin, ground
- 1 tablespoons coconut aminos
- 4 eggs
- ½ avocado, peeled, cored and chopped
- 1 tablespoon parsley, chopped

Directions:

In a fry pan, heat the ghee on medium-high heat and add the onions, jalapeno and garlic stirring and cooking until 3 mins. Add the meat, salt and pepper. Stir and cook for another 5 minutes. Stir in the cauliflower to cook 2 mins. Include sunflower seed butter, mayo, water, aminos, cumin. Mix and cook for another 5 minutes. Create four holes in this mix, break an egg into each hole, then Sprinkle with pepper and salt, then place the mix in the preheated oven and cook for 10 minutes. Divide this mixture between plates, sprinkle it with parsley, add avocado pieces to serve.

Enjoy!

Nutrition: calories 288, fat 12, fiber 6, carbs 15, protein 38

Zesty Zucchini Bread with Nuts

Ingredients for 4 servings
- 4 eggs
- 2/3 cup coconut flour
- 2 tsp baking powder
- 1 cup butter, softened
- 1 cup erythritol
- 2/3 cup ground almonds
- 1 lemon, zested and juiced
- 1 cup finely grated zucchini
- 1 cup whipped cream
- 1 tbsp chopped hazelnuts

Directions and Total Time: approx. 50 min + cooling time

Preheat the oven to 380 F. Grease a spring form pan and then line it with parchment paper. Set aside. Put the ingredients in a bowl and mix with erythritol and butter until smooth and pale. Add the eggs one at a time while whisking. Add baking powder and coconut flour and stir in the ground almonds, lemon zest, juice and zucchini. Pour the mix into the cake pan. The cake should bake for about 40 mins or till it is it has risen and a toothpick inserted in the cake is clean. Cool in it for about 10 minutes. Transfer the pan to the wire rack. Spread the whipped cream over and then sprinkle with hazelnuts. Serve and take pleasure in the delicious!

Per serving: Cal 804; Net Carbs 5g, Fat 83g; Protein 12g

Bell Peppers and Avocado Bowls

Ingredients for 4 servings:
- 2 tablespoons olive oil
- 2 shallots, chopped
- 1 red bell pepper, cut into strips
- 1 yellow bell pepper, cut into strips
- 1 green bell pepper, cut into strips
- 1 big avocado, peeled, pitted, and cut into wedges
- 1 teaspoon sweet paprika
- ½ cup vegetable stock
- Salt and black pepper to the taste
- 1 tablespoon chives, chopped

Instructions: (10 minutes preparation time, 15 minutes cooking time):

Heat up a pan with the oil medium heat, add the shallots and saute them for 2 minutes. Add the bell peppers and avocados and the other ingredients, excluding the chives. Toss and bring to a boil and cook on medium temperature for another 13 minutes. Mix the chives and toss the mixture, divide into bowls and serve with breakfast.

Nutrition: calories 194, fat 17.1, fiber 4.9, carbs 11.5, protein 2

Bacon, Cheese & Avocado Mug Cakes

Ingredients for 2 servings
- 2 eggs
- ¼ cup flax meal
- 2 tbsp buttermilk
- 2 tbsp pesto
- ¼ cup almond flour
- Salt and black pepper to taste
- 2 tbsp ricotta cheese
- 2 oz bacon, sliced
- 1 avocado, sliced

Directions and Total Time: approx. 15 minutes

Mix eggs, buttermilk and pesto together in the bowl of a food processor. Sprinkle with salt and pepper. Mix in the flax meal and almond flour, divide the mixture among 2 ramekins greased. Put them in the microwave and cook for about 2 minutes. Allow to cool before filling. In a nonstick skillet on medium-high heat, cook the bacon until crisp, approximately 5 minutes. Remove from heat and set aside. Transfer the ramekins onto plates and cut them in half across the middle. Sandwiches can be assembled by spreading ricotta on the top, and topping with avocado and bacon slices.

Per serving: Cal 528; Net Carbs 6.9g; Fat 44g; Protein 20g

Breakfast Bread

Preparation time: 10 minutes

Cooking time: 3 minutes

Servings: 4

Ingredients:
- ½ teaspoon baking powder
- ⅓ cup almond flour
- 1 egg, whisked
- A pinch of salt
- 2½ tablespoons coconut oil

Directions:

Grease a large microwave-safe mug with oil. In a bowl, mix eggs with flour and salt. Add oil along with baking powder. Place the mix in a mug and bake in a microwave for three minutes on high. Allow the bread to cool before removing it from the mug, cut into slices and serve.

Nutritional Value: Calories – 343, Fat – 38.5, Fiber – 0.4, Carbs – 0.8, Protein – 2.1

Pumpkin & Zucchini Bread

Ingredients for 4 servings
- 1 cup pumpkin, shredded
- 1 cup zucchini, shredded
- 1/3 cup coconut flour
- 6 eggs
- 1 tbsp olive oil
- ¾ tsp baking soda

- 1 tbsp cinnamon powder
- ½ tsp salt
- ½ cup buttermilk
- 1 tsp apple cider vinegar

Directions and Total Time: approx. 60 minutes

Preheat the oven to 360 F. In the bowl, combine all the ingredients and mix to create the dough. Place the batter in an oven-proof loaf pan that has been greased then bake it for about 45 minutes, or until the toothpick is clean. Allow to cool in the pan for five minutes. Serve the slices.

Per serving: Cal 185; Net Carbs 5g; Fat 13g; Protein 10g

Eggs and Sausages

Preparation time: 10 minutes

Cooking time: 35 minutes

Servings: 6

Ingredients:

- 5 tablespoons butter
- 12 eggs
- Salt and ground black pepper, to taste
- 1 ounce spinach, torn
- 12 ham slices
- 2 sausages, chopped
- 1 onion, peeled and chopped
- 1 red bell pepper, seeded and chopped

Directions:

In a skillet, heat 1 tablespoon butter on medium-high heat. Add onions, sausages stir, then cook 5 mins. In the meantime, add bell peppers and salt, stir and cook for about 3 minutes before transferring to the bowl. The rest of the butter should be melted and divide in 12 molds for cupcakes. Add one slice of ham in each mold, then divide spinach between them and mix in the sausage mixture. Sprinkle an egg on top, put in the oven, and bake at 425°F in 20 mins. Cool them briefly before serving.

Nutrition: Calories – 378, Fat – 28,4, Fiber – 1,5, Carbs – 6,2, Protein – 24,5

Ham & Cheese Sandwiches

Ingredients for 2 servings

- 4 eggs
- ½ tsp baking powder
- 5 tbsp butter, softened
- 4 tbsp almond flour
- 2 tbsp psyllium husk powder
- 2 slices mozzarella cheese
- 2 slices smoked ham

Directions and Total Time: approx. 20 minutes

For the creation of buns mix almond flour, baking powder, baking powder, 4 tbsp butter, egg and husk powder in a bowl. Mix until the dough is formed. Place the batter in two oven-proof mugs and microwave for 2 minutes or until firm. Remove the buns, flip them over, let them cool, then cut them in half. Place slices from mozzarella cheese and a piece of ham on one bun and then top it with the second. Warm the rest of the butter in a pan. Grill sandwiches until cheese has melted. Enjoy and serve!

Per serving: Cal 616; Net Carbs 4g; Fat 55g; Protein 30g

Avocados Stuffed With Salmon

Preparation time: 10 minutes

Cooking time: 0 minutes

Servings: 2

Ingredients:
- 1 big avocado, pitted and halved
- 2 ounces smoked salmon, flaked
- Juice of 1 lemon
- 2 tablespoons olive oil
- 1 ounce goat cheese, crumbled
- A pinch of salt and black pepper

Directions:

Using your food processor mix the salmon with oil, lemon juice, salt, and pepper. Pulse thoroughly. Divide the mix into avocado halves and serve.

Nutrition: calories 300m fat 15, fiber 5, carbs 8, protein 16

Almond & Raspberries Cakes

Ingredients for 4 servings
- 2 cups almond flour
- 2 tsp baking soda

- 1 tsp vanilla extract
- 2 tbsp almond flakes
- ½ tsp salt
- 2 tbsp liquid stevia
- 8 oz cream cheese, softened
- ¼ cup butter, melted
- 1 egg
- 10 raspberries
- 1 cup almond milk

Directions and Total Time: approx. 35 minutes

Mash the raspberries with a fork and set aside. Mix the almond flour, baking soda, vanilla, and salt in a large bowl. In a separate bowl, whisk the egg and almond milk. Add in the cream cheese, stevia, and butter and beat until well incorporated. Fold in the flour and mashed raspberries and spoon the batter into greased muffin cups two-thirds way up. Top with almond flakes. Bake for 20 minutes at 400 F until golden brown, remove to a wire rack to cool slightly for 5 minutes before serving.

Per serving: Cal 353; Net Carbs 5.6g; Fat 33g; Protein 10g

Spinach and Eggs Salad

Ingredients for 4 servings:
- 2 cups baby spinach
- 1 cup cherry tomatoes, cubed
- 1 tablespoon chives, chopped
- 4 eggs, hard boiled, peeled and roughly cubed
- Salt and black pepper to the taste
- 1 tablespoon lime juice
- 1 tablespoon olive oil

Instructions: (5 minutes preparation time, 0 minutes cooking time):

In a bowl, combine the spinach with the tomatoes and the other ingredients, toss and serve for breakfast right away.

Nutrition: calories 107, fat 8, fiber 0.9, carbs 3.6, protein 6.4

Bacon & Blue Cheese Cups

Ingredients for 4 servings
- 2 tbsp olive oil
- 6 eggs

- 2 tbsp coconut milk
- Salt and black pepper to taste
- ½ cup blue cheese, crumbled
- 4 oz bacon, chopped
- 2 tbsp chives, chopped
- 1 serrano pepper, minced

Directions and Total Time: approx. 30 minutes

Preheat oven to 390 F. Beat the eggs in a bowl and whisk in coconut milk until combined. Season with salt and pepper; fold in the blue cheese. Grease muffin cups with olive oil and spread the bottom of each one with bacon. Fill each with the egg mixture two-thirds way up. Top with serrano pepper and bake in the oven for 18 minutes or until golden. Remove and allow cooling for a few minutes. Serve topped with chives.

Per serving: Cal 414; Net Carbs 4.5g; Fat 34g; Protein 24g

Breakfast Muffins

Preparation time: 10 minutes

Cooking time: 30 minutes

Servings: 4

Ingredients:
- ½ cup almond milk
- 6 eggs
- 1 tablespoon coconut oil
- Salt and ground black pepper, to taste
- ¼ cup kale, chopped
- 8 prosciutto slices
- ¼ cup fresh chives, chopped

Directions:

In a bowl, mix eggs with salt, pepper, milk, chives, and kale. Grease a muffin tray with melted coconut oil, line with prosciutto slices, pour egg mixture, place in an oven, and bake at 350ºF for 30 minutes. Transfer muffins to a platter, and serve.

Nutritional Value: Calories – 257, Fat – 19.5, Fiber – 0.8, Carbs – 3.4, Protein – 18.1

Sesame & Poppy Seed Bagels

Ingredients for 4 servings
- ½ cup coconut flour
- 6 eggs
- ½ cup flaxseed meal

- ½ tsp onion powder
- ½ tsp garlic powder
- 1 tsp dried oregano
- 1 tsp sesame seeds
- 1 tsp poppy seeds

Directions and Total Time: approx. 30 minutes

Mix the coconut flour, eggs, ½ cup of water, flaxseed meal, onion powder, garlic powder, and oregano. Spoon the mixture into a greased donut tray. Sprinkle with poppy seeds and sesame seeds. Bake the bagels for 20 minutes at 360 F. Let cool for 5 minutes before serving.

Per serving: Cal 431; Net Carbs 3.3g; Fat 24g; Protein 20g

Scrambled Eggs

Preparation time: 10 minutes

Cooking time: 10 minutes

Servings: 1

Ingredients:

- 4 bell mushrooms, chopped
- 3 eggs, whisked
- Salt and ground black pepper, to taste
- 2 ham slices, chopped
- ¼ cup red bell pepper, seeded and chopped
- ½ cup spinach, chopped
- 1 tablespoon coconut oil

Directions:

In a pan, heat half the oil on medium-high heat. Add mushrooms and bacon, spinach, bell pepper and stir and cook for four minutes. Heat another pan with the remaining oil at medium-high temperature, add eggs and scramble them. Add the vegetables, ham, pepper and salt Mix and cook for one minute and serve.

Nutrition: Calories – 430, Fat – 31,9, Fiber – 2,4, Carbs – 9, Protein – 29,5

Nut Porridge with Strawberries

Ingredients for 2 servings
- 6 fresh strawberries, halved
- 4 tbsp chopped walnuts
- 2 tbsp chopped pecans

- 2 tbsp coconut flour
- 1 tsp psyllium husk powder
- 6 tbsp heavy whipping cream
- 2 oz butter
- 2 eggs
- 2 tbsp lemon juice
- 1 tsp cinnamon powder

Directions and Total Time: approx. 20 minutes

Place a saucepan over low heat. Mix with the flour and psyllium whipping cream, eggs, lemon juice and cinnamon in a bowl. Mix until well-combined. Add the mixture to the saucepan and cook for 10 mins and simmer, continuously stirring but don't boil until it becomes thick. Serve with strawberries, walnuts, pecans, and walnuts.

Per serving: Cal 650; Net Carbs 5.9g; Fat 60g; Protein 11g

Nutritious Breakfast Salad

Preparation time: 10 minutes

Cooking time: 6 minutes

Servings: 2

Ingredients:
- 3 cups kale, torn
- 1 teaspoon red vinegar
- A pinch of salt and black pepper
- 2 teaspoons olive oil
- 2 eggs
- 4 strips bacon, chopped
- 10 cherry tomatoes, halved
- 2 ounces avocado, pitted, peeled and sliced

Directions:

Place some water in a pot, bring it up to an unbeatable boil on moderate-high heat. Add eggs, boil them for six minutes, drain them, wash them and let them cool down by peeling and cutting the eggs. In a salad bowl mix the kale with vinegar and salt, pepper, oil, bacon, eggs, tomatoes and avocado. Toss them well. Divide the salad between plates and serve as breakfast.

Nutrition: calories 292, fat 14, fiber 7, carbs 18, protein 16

Cheesy Coconut Cookies

Ingredients for 4 servings

- ½ cup grated Gruyere cheese
- 1/3 cup coconut flour
- ¼ tsp baking powder
- ¼ cup coconut flakes
- 4 eggs
- ¼ cup butter, melted
- ¼ tsp salt
- ½ tsp xanthan gum
- 2 tsp garlic powder
- ¼ tsp onion powder

Directions and Total Time: approx. 35 minutes

Preheat the oven up to 350 F. Line a baking sheet with parchment paper. In the food processor, blend eggs and butter and salt until it is smooth. In a food processor, add coconut flour, xanthan gum, baking powder onion and garlic powders, and Gruyere cheese. Stir to blend. Form 12 balls from the mixture, and then place these on the baking sheets in 2-inch intervals. Bake for about 25 to 30 minutes, or till the cookies have a golden brown color. Allow to cool before serving.

Per serving: Cal 339; Net Carbs 5g, Fat 26g, Protein 11g

Creamy Eggs

Ingredients for 4 servings:

- 8 eggs, whisked
- 2 spring onions, chopped
- 1 tablespoon olive oil
- ½ cup heavy cream
- Salt and black pepper to the taste
- ½ cup mozzarella, shredded
- 1 tablespoon chives, chopped

Instructions: (10 minutes preparation time, 15 minutes cooking time):

In a pan, heat the oil on medium temperature, add spring onions and toss and cook them for three minutes. Add the eggs beaten with the cream and salt and pepper, and incorporate into the pan. Sprinkle the mozzarella on top of the mixture, cook it for 12 minutes, then divide the mixture between plates, then sprinkle the chives over it and serve.

Nutrition: calories 220, fat 18.5, fiber 0.2, carbs 1.8, protein 12.5

Spiced Biscuits

Ingredients for 4 servings

- 2 tbsp butter, melted
- ½ tsp baking soda
- 1 cup almond flour
- 1 egg
- ½ tsp salt
- ¼ tsp black pepper
- ¼ tsp garlic powder
- ½ tsp paprika powder
- ½ tbsp plain vinegar
- ½ cup mixed dried herbs

Directions and Total Time: approx. 35 minutes

Preheat the oven up to 350 F. Line a baking sheet with wax paper. In a bowl mix the flour, eggs, butter, salt, pepper, baking soda, garlic powder, vinegar, paprika and dried herbs. Stir until it is well-mixed. Make 12 balls of the mix and place them on the baking sheet in 2 inches intervals. Bake for 25 minutes or until golden brown.

Per serving: Cal 69; Net Carbs 0.6g, Fat 7g, Protein 1.5g

Vegetable Breakfast Bread

Preparation time: 10 minutes

Cooking time: 25 minutes

Servings: 7

Ingredients:

- 1 cauliflower head, separated into florets
- ½ cup fresh parsley, chopped
- 1 cup spinach, torn
- 1 onion, peeled and chopped
- 1 tablespoon coconut oil
- ½ cup pecans, ground
- 3 eggs
- 2 garlic cloves, peeled and minced
- Salt and ground black pepper, to taste

Directions:

In the food processor, mix cauliflower florets, salt and pepper and process until smooth. Cook a pan in oil on medium-low temperature, add the onions, cauliflower, garlic, a bit of spice and salt. Stir and cook for about 10 minutes. In a bowl mixing eggs with salt pepper, parsley, nuts, spinach and stir. Mix the cauliflower with the mixture and mix well. Form the mixture into shapes and place on a baking tray and then heat oven to 350 F, then cook for about 15 mins. Serve warm.

Nutritional Value: Calories – 105, Fat – 8.2, Fiber – 2.2, Carbs – 5.2, Protein – 4.2

Berry Hemp seed Breakfast

Ingredients for 2 servings

- ½ cup berry medley
- 1 cup coconut milk
- ¼ tsp vanilla extract
- 4 oz heavy cream
- 2 tbsp hemp seeds
- 4 tsp liquid stevia
- 1 tbsp sugar-free maple syrup

Directions and Total Time: approx. 10 min + cooling time

Mash the berries using a fork until it pureed them in the medium bowl. Add the coconut milk, hemp seeds, heavy cream vanilla, vanilla, and liquid Stevia. Mix well and chill the pudding over night. Serve the pudding in serving glasses, then top with maple syrup and serve.

Per serving: Cal 532; Net Carbs 7g; Fat 46g; Protein 10g

Frittata

Preparation time: 10 minutes
Cooking time: 1 hour
Servings: 4

Ingredients:

- 9 ounces spinach
- 12 eggs
- 1 ounce pepperoni
- 1 teaspoon garlic, minced
- Salt and ground black pepper, to taste
- 5 ounces mozzarella cheese, shredded
- ½ cup Parmesan cheese, grated
- ½ cup ricotta cheese
- 4 tablespoons olive oil
- A pinch of nutmeg

Directions:

Take the liquid from the spinach and place it in the bowl. In a separate bowl mixing eggs, add salt, pepper, nutmeg, garlic and whisk. In a third bowl, add spinach, Parmesan cheese, and the ricotta and whisk. Place the mix in a pan and sprinkle pepperoni and mozzarella cheese over it, bake in the oven baking at 375 F for about 45 minutes. Allow frittata to cool for a couple of minutes prior to serving.

Nutrition: Calories – 525, Fat – 40,7, Fiber – 1,4, Carbs – 6,7, Protein – 35,9

Morning Chia Pudding

Ingredients for 2 servings
- 2 tbsp chia seeds
- ¾ cup coconut milk
- 1 tbsp chopped walnuts
- ½ tsp vanilla extract
- ½ cup blueberries

Directions and Total Time: approx. 10 min + chilling time

Put the coconut milk, the vanilla as well as half the blueberries in blender. Blend all the ingredients until the blueberries are mixed in the mixture. Add the Chia seeds. Divide the mixture among two jars, cover and then refrigerate for four hours so that it can become gel. Add the black walnuts and blueberries. Serve.

Per serving: Cal 299; Net Carbs 7g; Fat 28g; Protein 9g

Breakfast Broccoli Muffins

Preparation time: 10 minutes
Cooking time: 30 minutes
Servings: 4

Ingredients:

- 2 teaspoons ghee, soft
- 2 eggs
- 2 cups almond flour
- 1 cup broccoli florets, chopped
- 1 cup almond milk
- 2 tablespoons nutritional yeast
- 1 teaspoon baking powder

Directions:

In a bowl mix the eggs, add the broccoli, flour and milk, yeast, and baking powder. Mix very well. Make muffins by rubbing a muffin tray using ghee. Divide the mixture of broccoli, then place to the oven, and bake to 350 degrees F in 30 mins. Serve

Nutrition: calories 204, fat 4, fiber 7, carbs 15, protein 11

Broccoli, Egg & Pancetta Gratin

Ingredients for 2 servings
- 10 oz broccoli florets
- 1 red bell pepper, chopped
- 4 slices pancetta, chopped
- 2 tsp olive oil
- 1 tsp dried oregano
- Salt and black pepper to taste
- 4 fresh eggs
- 4 tbsp Parmesan cheese

Directions and Total Time: approx. 30 minutes

Preheat oven to 420 F. Line a baking sheet with wax paper. Warm the olive oil in a pan over medium heat and stir-fry the pancetta for 3 minutes. Place the bell pepper, broccoli and pancetta on the baking sheet and stir together. Add salt, oregano and pepper. Cook for about 10 minutes or until the vegetables are soft. Remove, make four indentation and then put an egg in each. Then sprinkle with Parmesan cheese. Return to oven for about 5-7 minutes, or until egg whites have firmness and the cheese begins to melt. Take the dish out of the oven, and then serve.

Per serving: Cal 464; Net Carbs 8.2g; Fat 30g; Protein 30g

Shrimp and Eggs Mix

Ingredients for 4 servings:
- 8 eggs, whisked   1 tablespoon olive oil
- ½ pound shrimp, peeled, deveined, and roughly chopped
- ¼ cup green onions, chopped
- 1 teaspoon sweet paprika
- Salt and black pepper to the taste
- 1 tablespoon cilantro, chopped

Instructions: (5 minutes preparation time, 11 minutes cooking time):

In a pan, heat the oil on medium temperature, add springs, onions, mix and saute in 2 mins. Add the shrimp, stir and cook for another 4 minutes. Include the eggs along with the paprika the salt, and pepper. Mix and cook for an additional 5 minutes. Divide the mixture among plates, then sprinkle the cilantro over and serve it for breakfast.

Nutrition: calories 227, fat 13.3, fiber 0.4, carbs 2.3, protein 24.2

French Toast with Berry Yogurt

Ingredients for 2 servings
- ½ cup strawberries, halved
- ½ cup raspberries
- 2 eggs
- 1 cup Greek yogurt
- 2 tbsp sugar-free maple syrup
- ¼ tsp cinnamon powder
- ¼ tsp nutmeg powder
- 2 tbsp almond milk
- 4 zero-carb bread slices
- 1 ½ tbsp butter
- 1 tbsp olive oil

Directions and Total Time: approx. 20 min + chilling time

In a bowl, mix the yogurt, maple syrup and some berries. Cool for one hour. In a different bowl, whisk eggs, cinnamon, nutmeg and almond milk. Set aside. Slice each slice of bread into 4 pieces. Heat the butter and olive oil in a skillet over medium heat. Dip each slice in the egg mixture and bake until both sides are crispy, around 5-6 minutes. Serve warm with yogurt and berries.

Per serving: Cal 401; Net Carbs 9g; Fat 26g; Protein 17g

Breadless Breakfast Sandwich

Preparation time: 10 minutes

Cooking time: 10 minutes

Servings: 1

Ingredients:

- 2 eggs
- Salt and ground black pepper, to taste
- 2 tablespoons butter
- ¼ pound pork sausage, minced
- ¼ cup water
- 1 tablespoon guacamole

Directions:

In a bowl, mix minced sausage meat with pinch of salt and pepper, and stir well. Make a patty out of the mix and set it on the work surface. Prepare a pan using 1 tablespoon butter on medium-high heat. Add sausage patty and fry for 3 minutes each side before transferring onto an oven-safe plate. Crack an egg in 2 bowls and whisk it with spice and salt. Then, heat a pan along with the remaining butter on medium-high temperature, put two biscuit cutters greased inside the pan and add one egg to each. In the same pan add water. Lower the heat, cover the pan cooking eggs three minutes. Transfer the egg "buns" onto paper towels and then drain the all grease. Place a sausage patties onto the egg "bun," spread guacamole on top, and then cover with another egg "bun".

Nutritional Value: Calories – 735, Fat – 66, Fiber – 0.5, Carbs – 1.7, Protein – 33.6

Seeded Morning Loaf

Ingredients for 6 servings

- 4 tbsp sesame oil
- 6 eggs
- 1 cup cream cheese, softened
- ¾ cup heavy cream
- ¾ cup coconut flour
- 1 cup almond flour
- 3 tbsp baking powder
- 2 tbsp psyllium husk powder
- 2 tbsp desiccated coconut
- 5 tbsp sesame seeds
- ¼ cup flaxseed meal
- ¼ cup hemp seeds
- 1 tsp ground caraway seeds
- 1 tbsp poppy seeds
- 1 tsp salt
- 1 tsp allspice

Directions and Total Time: approx. 55 minutes

Preheat the oven at 350 F. In a bowl mixing almond and coconut flours, baking soda, psyllium husks, desiccated coconut, sesame seeds, flaxseed meal, hemp seeds, ground caraway seeds, poppy seeds, salt and all spice. In another bowl, mix eggs, heavy cream, cream cheese along with sesame oils. Combine the dry ingredients and blend all ingredients into a well-mixed dough. Place the dough in an oil-sprayed loaf pan. It should bake for approximately 45 minutes. Transfer onto a rack and let it cool.

Per serving: Cal 511; Net Carbs 4.7g; Fat 48g; Protein 21g

Chicken Breakfast Muffins

Preparation time: 10 minutes

Cooking time: 1 hour

Servings: 3

Ingredients:

- ¾ pound chicken breast, boneless
- Salt and ground black pepper, to taste
- ½ teaspoon garlic powder
- 1 tbsp cayenne pepper powder mixed with 3 tablespoons melted coconut oil
- 6 eggs
- 2 tablespoons green onions, chopped

Directions:

Sprinkle the chicken breasts by mixing salt, black pepper and garlic powder. Spread on a baking sheet lined with parchment and bake at 425 F for about 25 minutes. Transfer the chicken breasts into an empty bowl, then shred it using a fork, then mix in half of cayenne pepper powder and coconut oil that is melted. Sprinkle with a coating, and put aside. In the bowl mixing eggs, add salt and pepper, as well as onion greens, as well as the rest of the pepper. Mix with oils and stir. Divide the mixture into muffin tray. Top each with chicken, shredded then place them in the oven at 350 F then bake 30 mins. Serve muffins hot.

Nutritional Value: Calories – 338, Fat – 20.6, Fiber – 0.2, Carbs – 1.3, Protein – 35.3

Rolled Smoked Salmon with Avocado

Ingredients for 2 servings

- 2 tbsp cream cheese, softened
- 1 lime, zested and juiced
- ½ avocado, pitted, peeled
- 1 tbsp mint, chopped

- Salt to taste
- 2 slices smoked salmon

Directions and Total Time: approx. 10 min + cooling time

Mash the avocado using a fork in the bowl. Add the cream cheese lime, juice zest, mint and salt , and mix well. Place each salmon piece in a piece of wrap and filled with cream cheese mix. Wrap the salmon in a ball and secure the ends by twisting. Then, let it sit for two hours in the refrigerator. Then remove the plastic then cut off the wraps at both ends and then cut rolls into 1/2-inch pieces. Serve.

Per serving: Cal 520; Net Carbs 3g; Fat 31g; Protein 50g

Smoked Salmon Breakfast

Preparation time: 10 minutes

Cooking time: 10 minutes

Servings: 3

Ingredients:

- 4 eggs, whisked
- ½ teaspoon avocado oil
- 4 ounces smoked salmon, chopped
- For the sauce:
- 1 cup coconut milk
- ½ cup cashews, soaked and drained
- ¼ cup green onions, chopped
- 1 teaspoon garlic powder
- Salt and ground black pepper, to taste
- 1 tablespoon lemon juice

Directions:

With a mixer, blend cashews and coconut milk with garlic powder and lemon juice, then blend thoroughly. Incorporate salt, pepper and green onions. Blend once more than transfer to a bowl, then put it in the fridge. In a saucepan, heat oil on medium-low heat, include eggs and whisk and cook until nearly done. Set the eggs under the broiler in the oven and cook until the eggs are cooked. Divide the eggs onto plates, then top with the salmon smoked serving the salad sauce the top.

Nutrition: Calories – 448, Fat – 37,3, Fiber – 2,7, Carbs – 13,1, Protein – 19,8

Cauliflower Bake with Dilled Mayo

Ingredients for 4 servings

- 10 oz cauliflower florets
- 2 tbsp butter, melted
- Salt and black pepper to taste
- 1 pinch red pepper flakes
- ½ cup mayonnaise
- ¼ tsp Dijon mustard
- 3 tbsp Pecorino cheese, grated
- 1 tbsp dill, chopped
- 1 tsp garlic powder

Directions and Total Time: approx. 40 minutes

Preheat the oven up to 400 F. Mix mayonnaise with garlic powder, mustard, dill and salt in one bowl. Save in the refrigerator. Combine the cauli florets, salt, butter along with the flake in a bowl until well-mixed. Then, place the cauli florets in an oven dish coated with oil. Then sprinkle with Pecorino cheese, and bake for about 25 minutes, or until the cheese is melted and golden brown on top. Take it off, allow to sit for 3 minutes, then serve with the dilled sauce.

Per serving: Cal 233; Net Carbs 5g; Fat 19g; Protein 6g

Breakfast Pork Bagel

Preparation time: 10 minutes

Cooking time: 40 minutes

Servings: 6

Ingredients:
- 1 yellow onion, chopped
- 1 tablespoon ghee
- 2 pounds pork meat, ground
- 2 eggs
- 2/3 cup tomato sauce
- A pinch of salt and black pepper
- 1 teaspoon sweet paprika

Directions:

Prepare a pan using the ghee at medium-high heat. Add onion stir, and cook for about 3-4 minutes. Then, in a large bowl mix the meat, sauteed onions, eggs, tomato sauce, salt, pepper, and paprika. Stir thoroughly and form 6 bagels by using your hands. Place the meat bagels on a baking sheet lined with parchment and bake by baking them in the oven, at 400° F in 40 mins. Divide the bagels among plates, and then serve as breakfast.

Nutrition: calories 300, fat 11, fiber 8, carbs 16, protein 12

Mini Raspberry Tarts

Ingredients for 4 servings

- For the crust
- 2 cups almond flour
- 1 tsp cinnamon powder
- 6 tbsp butter, melted
- 1/3 cup xylitol
- For the filling
- ¼ cup butter,
- melted 3 cups raspberries,
- mashed ½ tsp fresh lemon juice
- ½ tsp cinnamon powder
- ¼ cup xylitol sweetener

Directions and Total Time: approx. 25 min + chilling time

Bake at 350 F. Lightly coat 4 mini tart tins of tart with cooking spray. Within a mixing bowl mix almond flour, butter with xylitol, cinnamon, and xylitol. Divide the dough into the tart tins and wait for fifteen minutes to bake. In a different bowl mix all the ingredients for the filling and stir to mix. Pour the filling into the pie and gently tap it on the flat surface to eliminate air bubbles, then chill for at least 1 hour.

Per serving: Cal 337; Net Carbs 5.6g, Fat 27g, Protein 2g

Garlicky Beef Bowls

Ingredients for 4 servings:
- 1 pound beef, ground   2 shallots, chopped
- 2 tablespoons tomato passata
- 1 green bell pepper, cut into strips
- 1 cup cherry tomatoes, halved
- 1 cup black olives, pitted and halved
- 1 tablespoon olive oil
- 2 green onions, chopped
- 3 garlic cloves, minced

- Salt and black pepper to the taste
- ½ tablespoon chives, chopped

Instructions: (10 minutes preparation time, 20 minutes cooking time):

In a pan, heat the oil on medium heat. Add the shallots, mix, then cook them for two minutes. In the meantime, add beef mix and cook for 5 minutes. Add the bell pepper along with the other ingredients. Toss and cook on medium temperature for another 12 minutes. Divide into bowls, and serve as breakfast.

Nutrition: calories 319, fat 14.4, fiber 3.3, carbs 10.3, protein 36.8

Spinach Nests with Eggs & Cheese

Ingredients for 2 servings
- 1 tbsp olive oil
- 1 tbsp dried dill
- 1 lb spinach, chopped
- 1 tbsp pine nuts
- Salt and black pepper to taste
- ¼ cup feta cheese, crumbled
- 2 eggs

Directions and Total Time: approx. 30 minutes

Saute the spinach in olive oil on medium temperatures for 5 minutes. Season with salt and black pepper and put aside. Prepare a baking sheet by coating it with cooking spray. Form two (firm and distinct) spinach nests onto the baking sheet and then crack an egg inside each nest. Decorate with feta and sprinkle with Dill. Bake for 15 minutes at 350 F just until the egg whites have set and the yolks are still runny. Serve the nests on plates decorated by pine nuts.

Per serving: Cal 308; Net Carbs 5.4g; Fat 22g; Protein 18g

Herbed Biscuits

Preparation time: 10 minutes

Cooking time: 15 minutes

Servings: 6

Ingredients:
- 6 tablespoons coconut oil

- 6 tablespoons coconut flour
- 2 garlic cloves, peeled and minced
- ¼ cup onion, minced
- 2 eggs
- Salt and ground black pepper, to taste
- 1 tablespoons fresh parsley, chopped
- 2 tablespoons coconut milk
- ½ teaspoon apple cider vinegar
- ¼ teaspoon baking soda

Directions:

In a bowl make a batter by mixing coconut flour, eggs, oil, garlic onions, coconut milk, salt, parsley and mix well. A bowl is used to mix the vinegar and baking soda. Stir thoroughly, then add it to batter. Scoop spoonfuls of the batter onto baking sheets that have been lined and then cut into circles. Place them in the oven at 350 F to 15 mins. Serve hot.

Nutritional Value: Calories – 213, Fat – 18.3, Fiber – 5.3, Carbs – 9.2, Protein – 4.1

Bacon & Mushroom "Tacos"

Ingredients for 2 servings
- 1 egg, hard-boiled and chopped
- 1 cup mushrooms, sliced
- 3 oz mozzarella cheese, grated
- 3 oz bacon, chopped
- 1 shallot, sliced
- 1 avocado, sliced
- 1 tbsp salsa
- 1 tbsp sour cream

Directions and Total Time: approx. 30 minutes

Pre-heat the oven to 350 degrees F. Set two piles of mozzarella cheese onto an oven dish lined with parchment and gently flatten with your hands to create taco shells (circle tortillas). Bake in the oven for 10-12 minutes until the edges brown; remove and let them cool slightly. Cook your bacon inside a skillet on moderate heat for about 4 minutes until crisp; transfer to an oven-safe bowl. Saute the shallot and mushrooms in the same grease for 5 minutes. Transfer from the bowl with bacon. Mix with eggs. Divide the mixture among the taco shells. Top with salsa, avocado and sour cream. Serve.

Per serving: Cal 563; Net Carbs 8g; Fat 48g; Protein 22g

Feta and Asparagus Delight

Preparation time: 10 minutes
Cooking time: 25 minutes
Servings: 2

Ingredients:

- 12 asparagus spears
- 1 tablespoon olive oil
- 2 green onions, chopped
- 1 garlic clove, peeled and minced
- 6 eggs
- Salt and ground black pepper, to taste
- ½ cup feta cheese

Directions:

Heat a pan with some water over medium heat, add asparagus, cook for 8 minutes, drain well, chop 2 spears, and reserve the rest. In a pan, heat oil at medium-low heat, add asparagus, garlic and onions, stir to cook, stirring for five minutes. Include eggs, salt and pepper mix, cover then cook 5 mins. Arrange asparagus spears over the frittata. Sprinkle cheese on top, bake at 350oF, then wait for about 9 minutes to bake. Divide the frittata among plates and enjoy.

Nutrition: Calories – 384, Fat – 28.3, Fiber – 3.4, Carbs – 9.7, Protein – 25.5

Roasted Stuffed Avocados

Ingredients for 2 servings
- 2 avocados, halved
- 3 eggs
- 1 tbsp Parmesan, grated
- Salt and black pepper to taste
- 1 tbsp parsley, chopped

Directions and Total Time: approx. 20 minutes

Scoop some of the avocado flesh into the bowl. Mash them with a fork. Then whisk into the eggs. Season by adding salt and pepper. Fill the avocado halves with the mixture and arrange them on a greased baking dish. Sprinkle with Parmesan cheese, and Bake in the preheated 350 F oven for about 8-10 minutes or until the eggs cook and cheese has melted. Garnish with fresh chopped parsley and serve.

Per serving: Cal 424; Net Carbs 4g; Fat 37g; Protein 14g

Easy Baked Eggs

Preparation time: 10 minutes

Cooking time: 20 minutes

Servings: 4

Ingredients:
- 1 cup baby spinach
- 4 ounces bacon, chopped
- 8 eggs, whisked
- A pinch of salt and black pepper

Directions:

Heat up a pan over medium-high heat, add bacon, stir and brown it for 4 minutes. Add baby spinach along with salt and pepper. Mix, cook for one minute longer, remove from the heat and divide into four ramekins. Divide whisked eggs within each ramekin, place them all into the oven, and bake to 400 degrees F over 15 minutes. Serve the eggs cooked to breakfast.

Nutrition: calories 281, fat 4, fiber 8, carbs 18, protein 6

Mushroom & Cheese Lettuce Cups

Ingredients for 2 servings
- 1 tbsp olive oil
- ½ onion, chopped
- Salt and black pepper to taste
- ½ cup mushrooms, chopped
- ¼ tsp cayenne pepper
- 2 fresh lettuce leaves
- 2 slices Gruyere cheese
- 1 tomato, sliced

Directions and Total Time: approx. 20 minutes

Warm the olive oil in a pan over medium heat. Saute the onion for 3 minutes, Cook the onion for 3 minutes until it becomes soft. Add the cayenne and mushrooms, and cook for 4-5 minutes, until soft. Add salt and pepper to taste. Pour the mixture of mushrooms into lettuce leaves. Top with cheese and tomato slices to serve.

Per serving: Cal 281; Net Carbs 5.7g; Fat 22g; Protein 12g

Tomato and Eggs Salad

Ingredients for 4 servings:

- 4 eggs, hard boiled, peeled and cut into wedges
- 2 cups cherry tomatoes, halved
- 1 cup kalamata olives, pitted and halved
- 1 cup baby arugula
- 2 spring onions, chopped
- A pinch of salt and black pepper
- 1 tablespoon avocado oil

Instructions: (5 minutes preparation time, 0 minutes cooking time):

Take a salad bowl mix the tomatoes, eggs and other ingredients. Toss, divide into smaller bowls, and serve as breakfast.

Nutrition: calories 126, fat 8.6, fiber 2.6, carbs 6.9, protein 6.9

Zucchini & Pepper Caprese Gratin

Ingredients for 4 servings
- 2 zucchinis, sliced
- 1 red bell pepper, sliced
- -Salt and black pepper to taste
- 1 cup ricotta cheese, crumbled
- 4 oz fresh mozzarella, sliced
- 2 tomatoes, sliced
- 2 tbsp butter
- ¼ tsp xanthan gum
- ½ cup heavy whipping cream

Directions and Total Time: approx. 50 minutes

Bake at 370 F. Make a layer of zucchinis and bell peppers into a greased baking dish overlapping. Sprinkle salt and pepper on top and then sprinkle with ricotta cheese. Repeat the layering process another time. Mix butter, xanthan Gum, as well as whipping cream, in microwave dishes for 2 minutes. Stir to combine completely, and sprinkle over the vegetables. Then, top with the remaining ricotta. Cook the gratin in oven for 30 mins or until the top is golden brown. Remove the gratin from the oven and layer it with fresh mozzarella and tomato slices. Bake for 5-10 minutes. Slice in pieces and then serve hot.

Per serving: Cal 283; Net Carbs 5.6g; Fat 22g; Protein 16g

Avocado Muffins

Preparation time: 10 minutes

Cooking time: 20 minutes

Servings: 12

Ingredients:

- 4 eggs
- 6 bacon slices, chopped
- 1 onion, peeled and chopped
- 1 cup coconut milk
- 2 cups avocado, pitted, peeled, and chopped
- Salt and ground black pepper, to taste
- ½ teaspoon baking soda
- ½ cup coconut flour

Directions:

Cook a pan on medium-high heat. Add onion, bacon, stir and cook for a couple of minutes. In a bowl, mash avocado pieces with a fork and whisk with eggs. Add salt, milk, baking soda, pepper and coconut flour and mix. Stir in the bacon mixture, and mix once more. Make a muffin tray greased with coconut oil, divide the avocado and eggs mixture in the tray, then place in the oven at 350 F. Bake in 20 minutes. Divide muffins onto plates and then serve.

Nutritional Value: Calories – 175, Fat – 15.1, Fiber – 2.6, Carbs – 4.8, Protein – 6.5

Arabic Poached Eggs in Tomato Sauce

Ingredients for 2 servings

- 4 large eggs
- ¼ cup yogurt
- 1 tsp olive oil
- 1 garlic clove, minced
- 1 small white onion, chopped
- 1 red bell pepper, chopped
- 1 small green chili, minced
- 1 cup diced tomatoes
- ½ cup tomato sauce
- 1 tsp cumin powder
- 1/3 cup baby kale, chopped
- ½ tsp dried basil
- ½ lemon, juiced Salt and black pepper to taste

Directions and Total Time: approx. 40 minutes

Warm olive oil in a deep skillet and saute garlic, onion, bell pepper, and green chili until softened, 5 minutes. Add tomatoes, tomato sauce and salt, pepper and cumin. Then cover and simmer for about 10 minutes. Include the kale, and cook until it is wilted. Add basil. Make four holes in the sauce using a wooden spoon. Then, crack an egg in each. Cover with a lid, and bake until eggs are set 8-10 minutes. Mix yogurt in a bowl and lemon juice. Serve the dish with the yogurt mixture and serve.

Per serving: Cal 319; Net Carbs 8g; Fat 17g; Protein 16g

Eggs Baked in Avocados

Preparation time: 10 minutes

Cooking time: 20 minutes

Servings: 4

Ingredients:

- 2 avocados, cut in half and pitted
- 4 eggs
- Salt and ground black pepper, to taste
- 1 tablespoon fresh chives, chopped

Directions:

Scoop out some of the flesh from the avocado halves and place in an oven-proof dish. Crack an egg into each avocado, sprinkle with salt and pepper and place in the oven at 425 F then bake it for about 20 mins. Sprinkle with chives towards the end, and serve.

Nutrition: Calories – 268, Fat – 24, Fiber – 6.7, Carbs – 9, Protein – 7.5

Tuna & Egg Salad with Chili Mayo

Ingredients for 4 servings

- 4 eggs
- 14 oz tuna in brine, drained
- ½ small head lettuce, torn
- 2 spring onions, chopped
- ¼ cup ricotta, crumbled
- 2 tbsp sour cream
- ½ tbsp mustard powder
- ½ cup mayonnaise
- ½ tbsp lemon juice

- ½ tbsp chili powder
- 2 dill pickles, sliced
- Salt and black pepper to taste

Directions and Total Time: approx. 20 minutes

Boil eggs with salted water at medium heat for eight minutes. Put them on an ice bath. Let cool, then chop them into smaller pieces. Transfer them into the bowl. Add the tuna, onions and mustard powder. Then add ricotta, lettuce, and sour-cream. Separately in a bowl mix the mayonnaise mixture, juice of a lemon and chili powder. Season according to your preference. Mix in the tuna mix and mix well. Serve with pickle slices.

Per serving: Cal 391; Net Carbs 4.5g; Fat 22g; Protein 35g

Eggs and Meat Patties

Preparation time: 10 minutes
Cooking time: 15 minutes
Servings: 4

Ingredients:
- ¾ pound pork, ground
- ¼ pound beef liver, ground
- ½ pound beef, ground
- 1 tablespoon maple syrup
- ½ teaspoon sage, dried
- ½ teaspoon rosemary, dried
- ½ teaspoon thyme, dried
- A pinch of salt and black pepper
- 4 eggs
- 2 tablespoons olive oil

Directions:

In a bowl mix the pork, beef, liver of the beef and sugar, maple syrup rosemary, thyme, salt and pepper. Stir and form four patties from this mixture. In a pan, heat half the oil on medium-high temperature, add the meat patties and make them cook for five minutes each side before dividing the patties between plates. Heat the same pan with the rest of the oil, crack the eggs, fry them, divide them next to the patties and serve for breakfast.

Nutrition: calories 342, fat 13, fiber 7, carbs 6, protein 34

Avocado Shakshuka

Ingredients for 2 servings
- 4 eggs
- 1 avocado, chopped
- 1 tbsp olive oil
- 1 medium red onion, sliced
- 1 zucchini, sliced
- 1 red bell pepper, sliced
- 1 yellow bell pepper, sliced
- 1 medium tomato, diced
- 1 cup vegetable broth
- 1 tbsp chopped parsley

Directions and Total Time: approx. 25 minutes

Heat your olive oil in a large skillet and saute the zucchini, onions, as well as bell peppers, for about 10 minutes. Add the tomatoes and broth. Bring to a boil, then reduce the heat until it becomes slightly thicker. Create four perforations in the sauce and place an egg in each of them. Let the eggs boil and then turn off the heat. Add avocado and parsley. Serve warm.

Per serving: Cal 448; Net Carbs 10g; Fat 39g; Protein 18g

Avocado Spread

Ingredients for 4 servings:
- 2 avocados, peeled, pitted, and chopped
- 1 tablespoon olive oil
- 1 tablespoon shallots, minced
- 1 tablespoon lime juice
- 1 tablespoon heavy cream
- Salt and black pepper to the taste
- 1 tablespoon chives, chopped

Instructions: (10 minutes preparation time, 0 minutes cooking time):

With a food processor, blend the avocado flesh, oils, shallots, and other ingredients, except for the chives. Pulse well. Divide into bowls, add the chives on top, and serve as a breakfast spread.

Nutrition: calories 253, fat 24.5, fiber 6.8, carbs 10.1, protein 2.1

Microwave Bacon Frittata

Ingredients for 2 servings

- 4 eggs
- 4 tbsp coconut milk
- ½ cup bacon, cubed
- ½ tsp oregano
- Salt and black pepper to taste
- 1 spring onion, sliced

Directions and Total Time: approx. 5 minutes

Within a bowl break eggs and beat them until they are combined. Season with black pepper and salt. Add bacon, coconut milk, spring onion, oregano and spring. Put the mix in two cups that are microwave safe. Microwave for one minute. Serve.

Per serving: Cal 370; Net Carbs 4.9g; Fat 27g; Protein 23g

Bacon and Lemon Thyme Muffins

Preparation time: 10 minutes

Cooking time: 20 minutes

Servings: 12

Ingredients:

- 1 cup bacon, diced
- Salt and ground black pepper, to taste
- ½ cup butter, melted
- 3 cups almond flour
- 1 teaspoon baking soda
- 4 eggs
- 2 teaspoons lemon thyme

Directions:

In a bowl make a mixture of flour, baking soda and eggs and mix thoroughly. Add lemon thyme, butter, bacon, salt and pepper. Whisk. Divide the mixture into a muffin pan lined with parchment and bake in the oven at 350 F. wait for 20 mins to bake. After cooling, the muffins can be divided into plates, and then serve.

Nutritional Value: Calories – 186, Fat – 17.1, Fiber – 0.8, Carbs – 1.8, Protein – 7.4

Lazy Eggs with Feta Cheese

Ingredients for 2 servings

- 4 eggs
- ¼ cup coconut milk
- ¼ cup feta cheese, grated
- 1 garlic clove, minced

- ¼ tsp dried dill
- ¼ tsp red pepper flakes

Directions and Total Time: approx. 10 minutes

Beat the eggs lightly using the fork in the bowl. Add the feta garlic, flakes and coconut milk. Divide the mixture into greased microwave-safe cups. The microwave should be on for 40 minutes. Mix well, then continue to microwave for another 70 minutes. Sprinkle with dill, and serve.

Per serving: Cal 234; Net Carbs 2.7g; Fat 16g; Protein 17g

Seasoned Hard Boiled Eggs

Preparation time: 10 minutes

Cooking time: 4 minutes

Servings: 12

Ingredients:

- 4 tea bags
- 4 tablespoons salt
- 12 eggs
- 2 tablespoons ground cinnamon
- 6star anise
- 1 teaspoon ground black pepper
- 1 tablespoon peppercorns
- 8 cups water
- 1 cup tamari sauce

Directions:

Place water in a pot, add eggs, bring to a boil at medium heat. Cook until they are hard-boiled. After cooling, crack them, without peeling. In a large saucepan make a mixture of water, tea bags and peppercorns, salt, cinnamon, peppercorns star anise, tamari sauce. Add the cracked eggs, cover pot, and bring to a simmer at a low temperature, to cook until 30 minutes. Remove tea bags, and simmer eggs for three hours and thirty mins. Allow the eggs to cool then peel them off and serve.

Nutrition: Calories – 122, Fat – 4.6, Fiber – 0.8, Carbs – 6.7, Protein – 13.9

Deli Ham Eggs

Ingredients for 2 servings

- 2 tbsp butter
- 1 shallot, chopped
- Salt and black pepper to taste
- 2 slices deli ham, chopped
- 4 eggs
- 1 thyme sprig, chopped
- ½ cup olives, pitted and sliced

Directions and Total Time: approx. 20 minutes

Beat the eggs gently with the help of a fork. Set the heat to medium, and then set the skillet with butter that is warm. Saute the shallots for 4 minutes until it is tender. Add the peppers, the ham and salt. Cook for another 5-6 minutes. Incorporate the eggs and garnish with the thyme. Cook for four minutes. Garnish with olives and serve.

Per serving: Cal 431; Net Carbs 6g; Fat 36g; Protein 21g

Cauliflower Cakes

Preparation time: 10 minutes

Cooking time: 20 minutes

Servings: 4

Ingredients:

- 1 cauliflower head, florets separated
- 2/3 cup almond flour
- 1 tablespoon nutritional yeast
- 2 eggs
- ½ teaspoon turmeric powder
- 2 tablespoons ghee
- A pinch of salt and black pepper

Directions:

Place the cauliflower florets into the pot, add enough water to cover the florets, bring to a boil at moderate heat. Cook for 8 minutes, then drain well. Place the cauliflower in your food processor, and blend well. A bowl is needed to mix all the ingredients: the eggs, flour yeast, salt, turmeric powder and pepper, combine well and make small patties from the mix. Prepare a pan using the ghee at medium-high temperature and add the patties. Cook for 3 minutes each side. Divide them into plates and serve them with breakfast.

Nutrition: calories 200, fat 3, fiber 8, carbs 16, protein 7

Serrano Ham Frittata with Salad

Ingredients for 2 servings
- 2 tbsp olive oil
- 3 slices serrano ham, chopped
- 1 tomato, cut into chunks
- 1 cucumber, sliced
- 1 small red onion, sliced
- 1 tbsp balsamic vinegar
- 4 eggs, beaten
- 1 cup Swiss chard, chopped
- Salt and black pepper to taste
- 1 green onion, sliced

Directions and Total Time: approx. 25 minutes

Whisk together vinegar, one teaspoon from olive oil, salt and pepper into a salad bowl. Add the tomatoes red onion, cucumber. Toss in a dressing. Sprinkle with serrano Ham. Heat the remaining olive oil in a pan over medium heat. Cook onions and Swiss Chard for three minutes. Sprinkle with salt and pepper cooking for two minutes. Pour the eggs on top the pan, turn down the heat to a simmer the cover, then let it cook on low for about 4 minutes. Transfer the pan into the oven. Bake the pan until golden on top in 5 mins in 390 F. Serve with sliced slices of the salad.

Per serving: Cal 354; Net Carbs 7g; Fat 26g; Protein 20g

Shrimp and Olives Pan

Ingredients for 4 servings:
- 1 pound shrimp, peeled and deveined
- 1 cup black olives, pitted and halved
- ½ cup kalamata olives, pitted and halved
- 2 spring onions, chopped
- 2 teaspoons sweet paprika
- 1 tablespoon olive oil
- Salt and black pepper to the taste
- ½ cup heavy cream

Instructions: (10 minutes preparation time, 10 minutes cooking time):

In a pan, heat the oil on medium heat. Add the onions, mix then cook them for two minutes. Add the shrimp and other ingredients, except for the cream, mix and cook for an additional 4 minutes. Then add the cream and mix with the shrimp, and cook on medium-high heat for another four minutes. Divide the mixture into plates and serve for breakfast.

Nutrition: calories 263, fat 14.8, fiber 1.7, carbs 5.5, protein 26.7

Goat Cheese Frittata with Asparagus

Ingredients for 2 servings
- 1 tbsp olive oil
- ½ onion, chopped
- 1 cup asparagus, chopped
- 4 eggs, beaten
- ½ habanero pepper, minced
- Salt and red pepper, to taste
- ¾ cup goat cheese, crumbled
- 1 tbsp parsley, chopped

Directions and Total Time: approx. 35 minutes

Pre-heat oven to 350 F. Saute the onion in olive oil on medium temperature until it is caramelized, about 6-8 minutes. Add the asparagus to the pan and simmer until soft, approximately 5 minutes. Add in habanero and eggs. Season with salt and red pepper. Cook until eggs are cooked. Sprinkle goat cheese and parsley over the frittata. Place in the oven to cook for 20 minutes or until the frittata is cooked to the middle. Cut into wedges prior to serving.

Per serving: Cal 345; Net Carbs 8.3g; Fat 37g; Protein 32g

Cheese and Oregano Muffins

Preparation time: 10 minutes
Cooking time: 25 minutes
Servings: 6

Ingredients:
- 2 tablespoons olive oil
- 1 egg
- 2 tablespoons Parmesan cheese

- ½ teaspoon dried oregano
- 1 cup almond flour
- ¼ teaspoon baking soda
- Salt and ground black pepper, to taste
- ½ cup coconut milk
- 1 cup cheddar cheese, grated

Directions:

In a bowl mix flour, oregano and salt, Parmesan cheese, and baking soda. In a different bowl mix coconut milk, olive oil, egg and stir it thoroughly. Combine the two ingredients and mix. Mix in cheddar cheese then pour the mix into the muffin tray lined with baking paper, and bake in the 350 F for about 25 minutes. Allow muffins to cool for a couple of minutes before you serve.

Nutritional Value: Calories – 204, Fat – 19.1, Fiber – 0.9, Carbs – 2.5, Protein – 7.6

Chorizo & Cheese Frittata

Ingredients for 2 servings
- 4 eggs Salt and black pepper to taste
- 1 chorizo sausage, sliced
- 1 tbsp butter
- 1 green onion, chopped
- ½ red bell pepper, crumbled
- 1 tsp chipotle paste
- ½ cup kale
- ¼ cup cotija cheese, shredded

Directions and Total Time: approx. 30 minutes

Whisk the eggs together in the bowl and then season with salt and black pepper. Heat butter in a pan at medium-low temperature. Saute the onion until it becomes soft. Add chorizo sausage chips, chipotle paste and bell pepper. Cook for 5-7 mins. In the kale, simmer for two minutes. Incorporate the eggs. Sprinkle the mixture evenly across the skillet, then place it in the oven. Cook for about 8 mins at 350 F to ensure the surface is cooked and golden. Sprinkle crumbled cotija cheese on top and bake for an additional 3 hours or till the cheese is completely melted. Serve the cheese slices while warm.

Per serving: Cal 435; Net Carbs 7.3g; Fat 31g; Protein 24g

Shrimp and Bacon Breakfast

Preparation time: 10 minutes
Cooking time: 15 minutes
Servings: 4

Ingredients:

- 1 cup mushrooms, sliced
- 4 bacon slices, chopped
- 4 ounces smoked salmon, chopped
- 4 ounces shrimp, deveined
- Salt and ground black pepper, to taste
- ½ cup coconut cream

Directions:

Heat a pan over medium heat, add bacon, stir, and cook for 5 minutes. Add mushrooms, stir to cook, and then simmer for five minutes. Add salmon, stir then cook 3 mins. Add shrimp, and boil for 2 mins. Sprinkle salt, pepper and coconut cream. Stir and cook for one minute remove from heat and place on plates.
Nutrition: Calories – 242, Fat – 16.8, Fiber – 0.8, Carbs – 2.9, Protein – 19.9

Bell Pepper & Cheese Frittata

Ingredients for 2 servings
- ½ green bell pepper, diced
- ½ cup feta cheese, crumbled
- 1 tomato, sliced
- 4 eggs
- 1 tbsp olive oil
- 2 scallions, diced
- 1 tsp dill, chopped
- Salt and black pepper to taste

Directions and Total Time: approx. 30 minutes

Preheat oven to 360 F. In a bowl, mix eggs with salt and pepper, until well-mixed. Add the bell peppers, cheese feta and scallions. Put the mix into an oven-proof casserole greased with oil, then garnish with tomato slices, then cook for about 20 minutes or until the frittata is cooked at the centre. Sprinkle with dill, and serve right away.

Per serving: Cal 421; Net Carbs 5.6g; Fat 35g; Protein 24g

Beef, Avocado and Eggs

Preparation time: 10 minutes
Cooking time: 11 minutes
Servings: 2

Ingredients:

- 8 mushrooms, sliced
- 1 yellow onion, chopped
- 1 tablespoon olive oil
- 3 ounces beef, ground
- A pinch of salt and black pepper
- 2 eggs, whisked
- ½ teaspoon smoked paprika
- 1 avocado, peeled, pitted and chopped
- 10 black olives, pitted and sliced

Directions:

In a skillet, heat the oil on medium-high heat and add the beef. Stir and cook for 4-5 mins. Add the onion and mushrooms, stir and cook for another 3 minutes. Add salt, pepper, paprika and eggs. Toss in the oven for 3-4 mins more, then divide into bowls, then top each bowl with olives and avocado and serve with breakfast.

Nutrition: calories 251, fat 4, fiber 8, carbs 14, protein 6

Crabmeat Frittata with Onion

Ingredients for 2 servings
- 1 tbsp olive oil
- ½ onion, chopped
- Salt and black pepper to taste
- 3 oz crabmeat, chopped
- 4 large eggs, slightly beaten
- ½ cup sour cream

Directions and Total Time: approx. 30 minutes

Set a pan on moderate heat and heat the oil. Sweat the onion until soft; place in the crabmeat and cook for 2 minutes. Sprinkle with salt and pepper. Distribute the ingredients at the bottom of the skillet. Mix the eggs using soy cream. Transfer the mixture into the skillet. Place the pan in the oven to cook for about 17 mins in a 350 F or until the eggs are cooked. Cut into wedges and serve.

Per serving: Cal 345; Net Carbs 6.5g; Fat 26g; Protein 23g

Pork and Avocado Mix

Ingredients for 4 servings:
- ½ cup tomato passata   1 pound pork, ground
- 1 avocado, peeled, pitted, and roughly cubed
- 1 tomato, cubed
- Salt and black pepper to the taste
- 8 eggs, whisked
- 2 spring onions, chopped
- 1 tablespoon avocado oil
- ½ teaspoon cayenne pepper
- 1 tablespoon chives, chopped

Instructions: (10 minutes preparation time, 22 minutes cooking time):

Heat a pan with the oil over medium heat, add the spring onions. Stir, and cook for 2 minutes. Add the meat, tomatoes and cayenne pepper. Toss and cook for 5 mins further. Add the tomato paste, the avocado eggs, salt and pepper. Toss and cook on medium heat for another 15 minutes. Divide into bowls, and serve as breakfast.

Nutrition: calories 431, fat 26.1, fiber 4.1, carbs 6.8, protein 42.3

Italian-Style Croque Madame

Ingredients for 6 servings
- 2 cups ricotta cheese
- 12 eggs
- 2 tbsp ground psyllium husk
- 2 tbsp coconut oil
- 8 oz Parma ham
- 3 oz mozzarella slices
- 1 red onion, chopped
- ½ cup basil leaves
- 1/3 cup toasted pine nuts
- ¼ cup grated Parmesan
- 1 garlic clove, peeled
- 6 tbsp olive oil

Directions and Total Time: approx. 30 minutes

In a food processor, puree basil, pine nuts, Parmesan cheese, garlic, and 4 tbsp of olive oil until desired consistency is reached; set aside the resulting pesto. In a bowl mix 8 eggs, the ricotta cheese and psyllium, husks until they are smooth and free of lumps. Let it sit for about 5 minutes. Warm the coconut oil in a skillet over medium heat. Pour a soup spoonful of mixture and place it in the pan and cook for two minutes on each side. Repeat with the rest of the batter. The pancakes should be spread half with pesto, then top them with cheese, ham, and onions. Layer the remaining pancakes. Heat the olive oil remaining in a skillet on moderate heat. Crack in the remaining eggs. Bake until whites have set but the yolks are soft and runny. Serve the eggs over the pancakes and garnish with pesto.

Per serving: Cal 584; Net Carbs 6g; Fat 48g; Protein 33g

Turkey Breakfast

Preparation time: 10 minute

Cooking time: 20 minutes

Servings: 1

Ingredients:
- 2 avocado slices
- Salt and ground black pepper, to taste
- 2 bacon slices, diced
- 2 turkey breast slices, already cooked
- 2 tablespoons coconut oil
- 2 eggs, whisked

Directions:

Heat a pan over medium heat, add bacon slices and cook throughout. In a second pan, heat oil on medium heat, add eggs, salt, and pepper and scramble. Slices of turkey breast bacon, scrambled eggs, bacon and avocado slices onto two plates, and then serve.

Nutritional Value: Calories – 791, Fat – 64.3, Fiber – 5.4, Carbs – 11.8, Protein – 41.8

Arugula Pesto Egg Scramble

Ingredients for 2 servings
- 1 tbsp butter
- 4 eggs
- 1 tbsp almond milk
- Salt and black pepper to taste
- Arugula pesto

- 1 cup arugula
- 1 cup Parmesan cheese, grated
- 1 tbsp pine nuts
- 1 garlic clove, minced
- ¼ cup olive oil
- 1 tbsp lime juice

Directions and Total Time: approx. 20 minutes

Beat eggs together in the bowl with the almond milk, salt and pepper. Place a skillet on medium-high heat, and heat the butter. Add the egg mixture and stir-fry until the eggs are set, but moist and tender. Set aside. In a blender, place all the ingredients for the pesto, excluding the olive oil. Pulse until smooth. As the blender is running, gradually add the olive oil until the desired consistency is achieved. Serve with the scrambled eggs and enjoy!

Per serving: Cal 592; Net Carbs 3.5g; Fat 53g; Protein 27g

Mexican Breakfast

Preparation time: 10 minutes
Cooking time: 30 minutes
Servings: 8

Ingredients:

- ½ cup tomato paste
- ½ tsp garlic powder
- 1 tsp dried basil
- 1 tsp dried oregano
- 1 tsp cumin
- 2 tsp chili powder
- 1 pound ground pork
- 1 pound chorizo, chopped
- Salt and ground black pepper, to taste
- 8 eggs
- 1 tomato, cored and chopped
- 3 tablespoons butter
- ½ cup onion, chopped
- 1 avocado, pitted, peeled, and chopped

Directions:

Mix in a bowl the spices and tomato paste for an enchilada sauce. In a different bowl mix the pork and chorizo. Stir, then place on a baking sheet. Sprinkle enchilada sauce over the top then place in the oven at 350 F, then wait for 20 minutes to bake. In a pan, melt butter on medium heat, add

eggs and then scramble them. Remove the pork mixture from the in the oven, and then spread scrambled egg mixture over the top. Sprinkle salt, pepper, tomato, avocado, and onion over the top, then divide it among plates, and then serve.

Nutrition: Calories – 513, Fat – 37.6, Fiber – 2.8, Carbs – 8.4, Protein – 35.6

Sausage Cakes with Poached Eggs

Ingredients for 2 servings

- ½ lb sausage patties
- 1 tbsp olive oil
- 2 tbsp guacamole
- ½ tsp vinegar
- Salt and black pepper to taste
- 2 eggs
- 1 tbsp cilantro, chopped

Directions and Total Time: approx. 20 minutes

Fry the sausage patties in warm olive oil over medium heat until lightly browned, 6-8 minutes. Transfer the sausage patties onto an uncooked plate. Then, spread the guacamole over. Boil the vinegar and two cups of water, in a saucepan at a high temperature, then reduce the temperature to simmer without boiling. Crack eggs into bowls and then gently place eggs into boiling water. Allow to simmer for a couple of minutes. Remove the egg from the water and place it onto a towel and let dry. Top each cake with a poached egg, sprinkle with cilantro, salt, and pepper and serve.

Per serving: Cal 583; Net Carbs 4.5g; Fat 43g; Protein 28g

Eggs and Tomato Sauce

Preparation time: 10 minutes
Cooking time: 30 minutes
Servings: 4

Ingredients:

- 1 tablespoon ghee
- 3 garlic cloves, minced
- 1 yellow onion, chopped
- 1 Serrano pepper, chopped
- 3 tomatoes, chopped
- 1 red bell pepper, chopped
- A pinch of salt and black pepper
- 1 teaspoon sweet paprika

- 1 teaspoon cumin, ground
- ¼ teaspoon chili powder
- 6 eggs

Directions:

Prepare a pan using the ghee on medium temperature; add onions and stir, then cook over 10 minutes. Add garlic, Serrano pepper, red bell pepper, a pinch of salt and black pepper, stir and cook for 10 minutes more. Add chili powder, tomatoes, cumin, paprika and cumin, mix and bring to a boil. Create 6 holes in the mix, break eggs in each one then cover the pan. Cook for another 10 minutes. Divide it among plates and serve it for breakfast.

Nutrition: calories 251, fat 5, fiber 8, carbs 17, protein 8

Morning Herbed Eggs

Ingredients for 2 servings
- 1 spring onion, finely chopped
- 2 tbsp butter
- 1 tsp fresh thyme
- 4 eggs
- ½ tsp sesame seeds
- 2 garlic cloves, minced
- ½ cup parsley, chopped
- ½ cup sage, chopped
- ¼ tsp cayenne pepper
- Salt and black pepper to taste

Directions and Total Time: approx. 15 minutes

Melt butter in a skillet over medium heat. Add garlic, parsley thyme, and sage. Stir-fry in 30-second intervals. Crack the eggs in the skillet. Reduce the heat and cook for 4-6 mins. The seasoning can be adjusted. If the eggs appear to be cooked, turn off the heat and transfer them to an eating plate. Serve the eggs with a drizzle of cayenne pepper and sesame seeds. Serve with spring onions.

Per serving: Cal 273; Net Carbs 4g; Fat 22g; Protein 13g

Beef Meatloaf

Ingredients for 6 servings:
- 2 shallots, chopped

- 1 tablespoon olive oil
- 1 green bell pepper, chopped
- 2 garlic cloves, minced
- 2 eggs, whisked   1 pound beef, ground
- Salt and black pepper to the taste
- 1 tablespoon cilantro, chopped

Instructions: (10 minutes preparation time, 45 minutes cooking time):

In a pan, heat the oil at medium-low temperature, then add the shallots and garlic mix, cook for five minutes. In a bowl, combine the shallots and garlic with the meat and the other ingredients, stir well, shape your meatloaf, and put it in a loaf pan. Place it in the oven to cook at the temperature of 380 degrees F for about 40 minutes. Cool the meatloaf and divide into plates and serve as breakfast.

Nutrition: calories 192, fat 8.6, fiber 0.3, carbs 2.5, protein 25.1

Scrambled Eggs with Tofu & Mushrooms

Ingredients for 4 servings
- 5 fresh eggs
- 1 tbsp butter
- 1 cup mushrooms, sliced
- 2 cloves garlic, minced
- 16 oz firm tofu, crumbled
- Salt and black pepper to taste
- 1 tomato, chopped
- 2 tbsp sesame seeds

Directions and Total Time: approx. 30 minutes

Melt the butter in a skillet over medium heat, and saute the mushrooms for 5 minutes until tender. Add the garlic, and cook for one minute. Mix the tofu into the dish and sprinkle by adding salt and pepper. Stir-fry for six minutes. Mix the tomatoes, and simmer, until soft over 5 minutes. Mix eggs together in the bowl before you pour them all on top of the tomato. Use a spatula immediately to stir the eggs until scrambled and not runny after 5 minutes. Add sesame seeds, and serve.

Per serving: Cal 385; Net Carbs 4.8g; Fat 27g; Protein 30g

Burrito

Preparation time: 10 minutes

Cooking time: 16 minutes

Servings: 1

Ingredients:

- 1 teaspoon coconut oil
- 1 teaspoon garlic powder
- 1 teaspoon cumin
- ¼ pound ground beef
- 1 teaspoon sweet paprika
- 1 teaspoon onion powder
- 1 onion, peeled, and julienned
- 1 teaspoon fresh cilantro, chopped
- Salt and ground black pepper, to taste
- 3 eggs

Directions:

Heat a pan over medium heat, add beef, and brown all over. Add salt and pepper, cumin, onion powder, garlic and paprika. Stir and cook for four minutes and then remove from the heat. In a bowl, mix eggs with salt, pepper, and whisk. Cook a pan in oil on medium-high temperature, add eggs then spread it evenly, and cook for six minutes. Transfer the egg burritos to an eating plate, then divide the beef mixture, add onions and cilantro, then roll and serve.

Nutritional Value: Calories – 482, Fat – 24.8, Fiber – 2.4, Carbs – 11.3, Protein – 52.2

Breakfast Pie

Preparation time: 10 minutes

Cooking time: 45 minutes

Servings: 8

Ingredients:

- ½ onion, peeled and chopped
- ½ red bell pepper, seeded and chopped
- ¾ pound ground beef
- Salt and ground black pepper, to taste
- 3 tablespoons taco seasoning
- ½ cup fresh cilantro, chopped
- 8 eggs
- 1 teaspoon coconut oil

For pie crust:

- 7 oz almond flour
- 2 oz coconut flour
- 1/2 tsp xanthan gum
- 1/2 tsp baking powder
- 6 oz butter (must be cold)
- 1 teaspoon baking soda

Directions:

Heat a pan with oil over medium heat, add beef, cook until it browns, and mix with salt, pepper, and taco seasoning. Stir again, then transfer to a bowl, and put aside. Cook the pan over medium heat. Add cooked juices of the beef, then add onions and bell pepper. Stir and cook for four minutes. Add baking soda, eggs, as well as salt, and mix thoroughly. Add cilantro, stir before removing the heat. In a large bowl mix pie crust ingredients. Store the mixture in the fridge for 1 hour. The pastry is then rolled, put an oven dish the pastry, and flip them up in the correct way. Place beef mixture in pie crust. Add vegetable mixture, spread on meat, then place in the oven that is set at 350 F to bake at least 45 minutes. Cool pie, cut into slices and divide into plates serving with papaya pieces.

Nutrition: Calories – 421, Fat – 34.8, Fiber – 2.7, Carbs – 6.3, Protein – 23.3

Bacon & Artichoke Omelet

Ingredients for 2 servings

- ¼ cup canned artichoke hearts, drained and chopped
- 4 eggs, beaten
- 1 tbsp heavy cream
- 4 bacon slices, chopped
- 1 tbsp olive oil
- 1 green onion, chopped
- Salt and black pepper to taste

Directions and Total Time: approx. 20 minutes

Warm the olive oil in a skillet over medium heat. Cook the bacon for 3 minutes. Add in the green onions, heavy cream and artichokes. Stir-fry for two minutes. Pour the eggs on top. Cook for 5-6 minutes, flipping once the omelet until the eggs are set. Season with salt and pepper. Serve.

Per serving: Cal 447; Net Carbs 3.3g; Fat 39g; Protein 19g

Chili Spinach and Beef Mix

Ingredients for 4 servings:

- 1 pound beef meat, ground
- 1 tablespoons avocado oil

- 2 shallots, chopped
- 2 garlic cloves, minced
- 2 teaspoons red chili flakes
- 1 tablespoon tomato passata
- 1 cup baby spinach
- 1 teaspoon chili powder
- Salt and black pepper to the taste

Instructions: (10 minutes preparation time, 26 minutes cooking time):

Prepare a pan using the oil on medium heat. Add the shallots, garlic. Stir, then cook 3 mins. Add the meat and cook the meat for five minutes. Add the chili powder and other ingredients, mix in the pan, and cook at medium-high temperature for 15 minutes, Divide into bowls, and serve as breakfast.

Nutrition: calories 239, fat 9.2, fiber 1.1, carbs 3.2, protein 34.1

Chili Omelet with Avocado

Ingredients for 2 servings
- 2 tsp olive oil
- 1 ripe avocado, chopped
- 2 spring onions, chopped
- 2 spring garlic, chopped
- 4 eggs
- 1 cup buttermilk
- 2 tomatoes, sliced
- 1 green chili pepper, minced
- 2 tbsp fresh cilantro, chopped Salt and black pepper to taste

Directions and Total Time: approx. 15 minutes

Crack eggs into the bowl, then whisk in buttermilk, salt along with black pepper. Set the pan on high heat and warm the olive oil. Saute onions and garlic until they are tender and translucent. Pour the mixture into the pan and make use of a spatula to smooth the surface. Cook until the eggs puff up and brown at the bottom. Include chili pepper, cilantro avocado, tomatoes, and chili pepper on the other side of the egg dish. Fold it in half, then cut into pieces. Serve immediately.

Per serving: Cal 422; Net Carbs 11g; Fat 32g; Protein 19g

Breakfast Hash

Preparation time: 10 minutes

Cooking time: 16 minutes

Servings: 2

Ingredients:
- 1 tablespoon coconut oil
- 2 garlic cloves, peeled and minced
- ½ cup beef stock
- Salt and ground black pepper, to taste
- 1 onion, peeled and chopped
- 2 cups corned beef, chopped
- 1 pound radishes, cut in quarters

Directions:

In a fry pan, heat the oil at medium-high and add onions, mix and cook for four minutes. Add radishes, stir then cook 5 mins. Add garlic, stir and cook for one minute. Add beef, stock, salt, pepper, stir and simmer for five minutes. Remove off the heat and serve.

Nutritional Value: Calories – 316, Fat – 21.2, Fiber – 4.9, Carbs – 13.9, Protein – 18

Bacon & Cheese Cloud Eggs

Ingredients for 2 servings

- 4 eggs, whites and yolks separated
- Salt and black pepper to taste
- 2 bacon slices
- 1 tbsp chives, finely chopped,
- 3 tbsp grated Pecorino cheese

Directions and Total Time: approx. 15 minutes

Heat a skillet over medium heat. Cook the bacon until crisp in both directions, approximately 5 minutes. Allow it to cool, then break it up. With an electric mixer mix the egg yolks with salt until stiff peak forms. Mix in your Pecorino cheese and bacon. Spoon the mixture into 4 mounds on a parchment-lined baking sheet. Create an indention in each pile. Carefully spoon an egg yolk into each indention; season with salt and pepper. Bake in the preheated to 450 F oven for 3 minutes until the yolks are set. Sprinkle with chives and serve.

Per serving: Cal 287; Net Carbs 4.7g; Fat 24g; Protein 12g

Breakfast Stir-fry

Preparation time: 10 minutes
Cooking time: 30 minutes
Servings: 2

Ingredients:

- ½ pounds minced beef
- 2 teaspoons red chili flakes
- 1 tablespoon tamari sauce
- 2 bell peppers, seeded and chopped
- 1 teaspoon chili powder
- 1 tablespoon coconut oil
- Salt and ground black pepper, to taste

For the bok choy:
- 6 bunches bok choy, trimmed and chopped
- 1 teaspoon fresh ginger, grated
- Salt, to taste
- 1 tablespoon coconut oil

For the eggs:
- 1 tablespoon coconut oil
- 2 eggs

Directions:

In a pan, heat 1 teaspoon coconut oil on medium-high heat. Add bell peppers, beef stir and simmer for about 10 minutes. Add salt, chili powder, pepper, tamari sauce, chili flakes, stir, cook for 4 minutes and remove from the heat. Heat another pan with 1 tablespoon oil over medium heat, add bok choy, stir, and cook for 3 minutes. Add ginger, salt stir and cook for 2 minutes and switch off the heat. Heat third pan with 1 tablespoon oil over medium heat, crack eggs into pan and fry them. Divide the bell pepper and beef mixture into two bowls. Divide the bok choy, and then garnish with eggs.

Nutrition: Calories – 510, Fat – 32.6, Fiber – 3.4, Carbs – 13.1, Protein – 43.4

Canadian Bacon Eggs Benedict

Ingredients for 2 servings
- 1 tsp white wine vinegar
- 2 large eggs

- 4 Canadian bacon slices
- 1 tbsp fresh parsley, chopped

Directions and Total Time: approx. 20 minutes

Heat a skillet over medium heat and fry the bacon for 3-4 minutes per side. Transfer to a towel to absorb the excess fat. Bring the vinegar and water to a boil in a saucepan over high heat. Then reduce it to simmer. Crack eggs into bowls and then gently place eggs into boiling water. Allow to simmer for a couple of minutes. Utilize a spoon with a perforated hole to scoop the egg from the water and place it on the newspaper towel and dry. Set the bacon on 2 plates. Top each with an egg. Sprinkle with parsley.

Per serving: Cal 161; Net Carbs 1.4g;Fat 9g; Protein 18g

Fast Scramble

Preparation time: 10 minutes
Cooking time: 10 minutes
Servings: 1

Ingredients:
- 4 mushrooms, chopped
- 3 eggs, whisked
- ¼ cup red bell pepper, chopped
- 1 tablespoon ghee, melted
- 2 bacon slices, chopped
- A pinch of salt and black pepper

Directions:

In a skillet, heat the ghee at medium-high and add bacon. Stir to cook 3-4 mins. Add the bell pepper and mushrooms stir, cook for another 3-4 minutes. Sprinkle salt, pepper and eggs. Stir to cook the eggs until scramble is cooked. Divide the scramble between plates, and serve with breakfast.

Nutrition: calories 200, fat 4, fiber 6, carbs 16, protein 7

Chorizo Egg Cups

Ingredients for 2 servings
- 1 tsp butter, melted
- 4 eggs, beaten

- Salt and black pepper to taste
- 1 cup mozzarella, grated
- 2 chorizo sausages, chopped
- 1 tbsp parsley, chopped

Directions and Total Time: approx. 20 minutes

In a bowl, stir the eggs, sausages, and cheese; season with salt and pepper. Pour the mixture into butter-greased muffin cups, then bake for 8 to 10 mins in the oven at 404 F. Sprinkle with parsley to serve.

Per serving: Cal 452; Net Carbs 2.4g; Fat 35g; Protein 31g

Zucchini Spread

Ingredients for 4 servings:
- 1 pound zucchinis, roughly cubed
- 1 cup heavy cream
- 2 shallots, chopped
- 1 tablespoon lime juice
- 1 tablespoon avocado oil
- Salt and black pepper to the taste
- 1 tablespoon basil, chopped

Instructions: (10 minutes preparation time, 17 minutes cooking time):

In a pan, heat the oil on medium-high temperature, add the shallots and stir and cook for 2 minutes. Add the zucchinis and the other ingredients, mix to cook at medium-low temperatures for about 15 minutes. Allow to cool, then transfer the mixture to the blender, and pulse it several times, then divide into bowls, and serve as a breakfast.

Nutrition: calories 240, fat 7.6, fiber 2, carbs 5.9, protein 11.2

Brussels Sprout Delight

Preparation time: 10 minutes

Cooking time: 12 minutes

Servings: 3

Ingredients:
- 3 eggs
- Salt and ground black pepper, to taste
- 1 tablespoon butter, melted

- 2 shallots, peeled and minced
- 2 garlic cloves, peeled and minced
- 12 ounces Brussels sprouts, sliced thin
- 2 ounces bacon, chopped
- 1½ tablespoons apple cider vinegar

Directions:

Heat a pan on medium heat. Add bacon stir and to cook till crispy. then transfer onto a plate and put aside. In the same pan, over medium heat, add shallots, garlic and shallots. Stir, simmer for about 30 seconds. Then add Brussels sprouts, salt and pepper and apple cider vinegar. Stir then cook 5 mins. Add bacon back to the pan, stir to cook, and then simmer for five minutes. Stir in butter and create a hole in the middle. Crack eggs in pan to cook them thoroughly. Then serve.

Nutritional Value: Calories – 275, Fat – 16.5, Fiber – 4.3, Carbs – 17.2, Protein – 17.4

Cereal Nibs

Preparation time: 10 minutes

Cooking time: 45minutes

Servings: 4

Ingredients:
- 4 tablespoons hemp hearts
- ½ cup chia seeds
- 1 cup water
- 1 tablespoon vanilla extract
- 1 tablespoon psyllium powder
- 2 tablespoons coconut oil
- 1 tablespoon swerve
- 2 tablespoons cocoa nibs

Directions:

In a bowl, mix the chia seeds in water. Mix, then stir and let it sit for five minutes. Add vanilla extract, hemp hearts and psyllium powder to mix well, swerve and stir well with the help of a mixer. Add cocoa nibs, and mix until you get the form of a dough. Divide the dough into two pieces, then shape into a cylindrical shape, place them on a baking tray lined with baking paper then flatten and cover with parchment paper, put in the oven at 285 F, and cook for about 20 mins. Remove parchment paper, bake for another 25 minutes. Take the cylinders out of the oven, allow to cool and then cut them into small pieces prior to serving.

Nutritional Value: Calories – 324, Fat – 25.4, Fiber – 8.1, Carbs – 14.3, Protein – 12.8

Breakfast Skillet

Preparation time: 10 minutes

Cooking time: 30 minutes

Servings: 4

Ingredients:

- 8 ounces mushrooms, chopped
- Salt and ground black pepper, to taste
- 1 pound minced pork
- 1 tablespoon coconut oil
- ½ teaspoon garlic powder
- ½ teaspoon dried basil
- 2 tablespoons Dijon mustard
- 2 zucchini, chopped

Directions:

In a pan, heat oil over medium-high heat, add the mushrooms, stir to cook, stirring for four minutes. Include zucchini with salt, and pepper Stir, then cook 4 mins. Add the pork and Basil, garlic powder, a pinch of salt and black pepper. Stir and cook until the meat is cooked. Mix in mustard and cook for 3 minutes. Divide into bowls and serve.

Nutrition: Calories – 225, Fat – 8, Fiber – 1.9, Carbs – 5.6, Protein – 33

Delicious Tomato Scramble

Preparation time: 10 minutes

Cooking time: 10 minutes

Servings: 2

Ingredients:

- 1 tablespoon coconut oil, melted
- 6 eggs, whisked
- 15 ounces canned tomatoes, chopped
- A pinch of salt and black pepper
- 2 tablespoons parsley, chopped

Directions:

Prepare a pan using the oil on medium-high heat and add tomatoes, salt and pepper. Mix and

simmer for four minutes. Add eggs to stir, cook for about 6 minutes until the scramble is ready. Divide the eggs between plates, sprinkle parsley over the top and serve with breakfast.

Nutrition: calories 201, fat 3, fiber 4, carbs 15, protein 7

Spinach Omelet

Ingredients for 4 servings:
- 8 eggs, whisked   1 cup baby spinach
- A pinch of salt and black pepper
- 1 tablespoon olive oil
- 2 spring onions, chopped
- 1 teaspoon sweet paprika
- 1 teaspoon cumin, ground
- 1 tablespoon chives, chopped

Instructions: (10 minutes preparation time, 20 minutes cooking time):

Prepare a pan using the oil on medium heat. Add spring onions along with the paprika, as well as cumin. Stir and cook for five minutes. Include the eggs spinach with salt and pepper, mix, then pour into the skillet, then cover with a lid and cook for 15 minutes. Sprinkle the chives over Divide everything among dishes and serve.

Nutrition: calories 345, fat 12, fiber 1.5, carbs 8, protein 13.3

Chia Pudding

Preparation time: 10 minutes

Cooking time: 30 minutes

Servings: 2

Ingredients:
- 2 tablespoons coffee
- 2 cups water
- ⅓ cup chia seeds
- 1 tablespoon swerve
- 1 tablespoon vanilla extract
- 2 tablespoons cocoa nibs
- ⅓ cup coconut cream

Directions:

In a small saucepan, heat water at a medium temperature and bring it to a boil, then add coffee and simmer for 15 minutes. Take off the heat and pour into an ice cube. Add vanilla extract, coconut cream and swerve cocoa nibs and chia seeds. Stir thoroughly, then store it in the fridge for at least 30 minutes, then divide into two breakfast bowls and serve.

Nutritional Value: Calories – 149, Fat – 12.5, Fiber – 2.9, Carbs – 10.8, Protein – 2

Hemp Porridge

Preparation time: 3 minutes

Cooking time: 3 minutes

Servings: 1

Ingredients:

- 1 tablespoon chia seeds
- 1 cup almond milk
- 2 tablespoons flaxseeds
- ½ cup hemp hearts
- ½ teaspoon ground cinnamon
- 1 tablespoon stevia
- ¾ teaspoon vanilla extract
- ¼ cup almond flour
- 1 tablespoon hemp hearts, for serving

Directions:

In a pan, mix almond milk with half cup of hemp heart, chia seeds flaxseeds and vanilla extract, cinnamon Mix well and cook on medium temperature. For two minutes, then remove from the heat, and mix in almond flour. Mix well and then pour into the bowl. Serve with 1 teaspoon hemp heart and serve.

Nutritional Value: Calories – 1030, Fat – 91.6, Fiber – 18.5, Carbs – 32.7, Protein – 29.5

Breakfast Casserole

Preparation time: 10 minutes

Cooking time: 40 minutes

Servings: 4

Ingredients:

- 10 eggs
- 1 pound pork sausage, chopped
- 1 onion, peeled and chopped
- 3 cups spinach, torn
- Salt and ground black pepper, to taste
- 3 tablespoons avocado oil

Directions:

In a skillet, heat 1 tablespoon of oil on medium heat. Add sausage, stir and cook it in 4 minutes. Add onion then cook it for three minutes. Add spinach, stir and cook for one minute. Grease a baking dish using the remaining oil, then pour the sausage mix in it. Whisk eggs before adding them to the sausage mix. Stir well, put in the oven at 350 F, then cook for about 30 mins. The casserole should rest for a few minutes prior to serving.

Nutrition: Calories – 572, Fat – 44.5, Fiber – 1.6, Carbs – 4.8, Protein – 36.9

Easy Frittata

Preparation time: 10 minutes

Cooking time: 15 minutes

Servings: 2

Ingredients:

- 1 tablespoon ghee, melted
- 4 eggs, whisked
- A pinch of salt and black pepper
- 1 shallot, chopped
- 4 cherry tomatoes, halved
- 4 prosciutto slices, chopped
- 2 garlic cloves, minced
- 2 tablespoons olive oil
- 1 tablespoon parsley, chopped

Directions:

In a bowl mix the chopped parsley, garlic and olive oil. Mix well before putting the bowl aside until later. Prepare a pan using the ghee at medium-low heat. Add shallot, stir and cook for two minutes. Add tomatoes, prosciutto and whisked eggs, and mix a little. Add salt and pepper, place to the oven and bake at 390 F in 10 mins. Divide the frittata among plates, pour the olive oil mixture over the top and serve it for breakfast.

Nutrition: calories 271, fat 4, fiber 7, carbs 18, protein 7

Sage Zucchini Cakes

Ingredients for 4 servings:

- 1 pound zucchinis, grated and excess water drained

- Salt and black pepper to the taste
- 1 tablespoon almond flour
- 1 egg, whisked
- 1 tablespoon sage, chopped
- 2 tablespoons olive oil

Instructions: (10 minutes preparation time, 12 minutes cooking time):

In a bowl, combine the zucchinis with the flour and the other ingredients except the oil, stir well and shape medium cakes out of this mix. Prepare a pan using oil on medium temperature, then add the cakes and cook for 5 to 6 minutes on each side. Drain the excess grease onto paper towels. Divide the cakes into plates, and serve for breakfast.

Nutrition: calories 320, fat 13.32, fiber 5.2, carbs 10, protein 12.1

Simple Breakfast Cereal

Preparation time: 10 minutes
Cooking time: 3 minutes
Servings: 2

Ingredients:
- ½ cup coconut, shredded
- 4 teaspoons butter
- 2 cups almond milk
- 1 tablespoon stevia
- A pinch of salt
- ⅓ cup macadamia nuts, chopped
- ⅓ cup walnuts, chopped
- ⅓ cup flaxseed

Directions:

In a saucepan, melt butter on medium heat. Add coconut milk, macadamia nuts, salt, flaxseed, walnuts and stevia. Stir thoroughly. After 3 minutes of cooking then stir, remove off the heat, and let it sit until 10 minutes. Divide the soup into two bowls and serve.

Nutritional Value: Calories – 1078, Fat – 106.6, Fiber – 15.5, Carbs – 26.8, Protein – 16.5

Simple Egg Porridge

Preparation time: 10 minutes

Cooking time: 4 minutes
Servings: 2

Ingredients:
- 2 eggs
- 1 tablespoon stevia
- ⅓ cup heavy cream
- 2 tablespoons butter, melted
- A pinch of ground cinnamon

Directions:

In a bowl make a mixture of eggs, heavy cream and stevia and then whisk. In a fry pan, melt butter over medium-high and add the egg mixture and cook until cooked. Transfer the mixture to two bowls, sprinkle some cinnamon on the top and serve.

Nutritional Value: Calories – 234, Fat – 23.3, Fiber – 0, Carbs – 0.9, Protein – 6.1

Sausage Patties

Preparation time: 10 minutes
Cooking time: 10 minutes
Servings: 4

Ingredients:
- 1 pound minced pork
- Salt and ground black pepper, to taste
- ¼ teaspoon dried thyme
- ½ teaspoon dried sage
- ¼ teaspoon ground ginger
- 3 tablespoons cold water
- 1 tablespoon coconut oil

Directions:

Put meat in a bowl. In a different bowl, mix water, salt pepper, sage, ginger, and thyme and then whisk. Add the mixture to the meat and mix thoroughly. Make patties and set them on a surface to work. Make a pan of coconut oil on medium-high heat and add the patties. Fry them for 5 minutes. Then flip and cook for another 3 minutes. Serve warm.

Nutrition: Calories – 191, Fat – 7.4, Fiber – 0, Carbs – 0, Protein – 29.7

Salmon Frittata

Preparation time: 10 minutes
Cooking time: 10 minutes
Servings: 2

Ingredients:

- ½ teaspoon avocado oil
- 4 ounces smoked salmon, skinless, boneless and chopped
- 4 eggs, whisked
- A pinch of black pepper
- 2 green onions, chopped
- 1 tablespoon parsley, chopped

Directions:
Prepare a pan using the oil on medium-high heat, add green onions along with black pepper and salmon. Stir and cook for around 3 minutes. Add whisked eggs, stir some then cover the pan and cook until the frittata has completed. Slice the frittata, divide it into plates. Sprinkle the top with parsley and serve it for breakfast.

Nutrition: calories 261, fat 4, fiber 7, carbs 17, protein 7

Pork Casserole

Ingredients for 4 servings:

- 1 pound pork, ground
- Salt and black pepper to the taste
- 2 shallots, chopped
- 2 garlic cloves, minced
- 1 tablespoon olive oil
- 2 red bell peppers, roughly cubed
- 2 tomatoes, cubed
- 1 cup mozzarella, shredded
- 2 tablespoons parsley, chopped

Instructions: (10 minutes preparation time, 45 minutes cooking time):

Prepare a pan using the oil at medium-low heat. Add the shallots and garlic, and cook for five minutes. Add the meat along with bell peppers and tomatoes. Stir and cook for another 5 minutes. Make an oven-proof casserole, sprinkle the mozzarella and parsley on top, bake into the oven to cook at 350 F at 35 minutes. Divide the mix among plates, and serve for breakfast.

Nutrition: calories 340, fat 28, fiber 5.3, carbs 6.3,

protein 17.6

Sausage Quiche

Preparation time: 10 minutes
Cooking time: 40 minutes
Servings: 6

Ingredients:

- 12 ounces pork sausage, chopped
- Salt and ground black pepper, to taste
- 2 teaspoons whipping cream
- 2 tablespoons fresh parsley, chopped
- 10 mixed cherry tomatoes, halved
- 6 eggs
- 2 tablespoons Parmesan cheese, grated
- 5 eggplant slices

Directions:

Place sausage pieces in baking dish. Place slices of eggplant on top and then add cherry tomatoes. In the bowl mix eggs, add salt, pepper, cream and Parmesan cheese. Whisk. Pour the mixture into the dish for baking, and place in the oven at 375 F. cook for about 40 mins and then serve.

Nutrition: Calories – 275, Fat – 21.5, Fiber – 0.4, Carbs – 1.9, Protein – 17.7

Rosemary Frittata

Preparation time: 10 minutes
Cooking time: 15 minutes
Servings: 4

Ingredients:

- 8 eggs, whisked
- 1 tablespoon avocado oil
- 1 tablespoon coconut cream
- 2 thyme springs, chopped
- 3 rosemary springs, chopped
- ¼ teaspoon cinnamon powder
- 2 garlic cloves, minced
- ¼ teaspoon nutmeg, ground
- ¼ cup hazelnuts, chopped
- A pinch of salt and black pepper

Directions:

Heat up a pan with the oil over medium heat, add

garlic, rosemary and thyme, stir and cook for 2-3 minutes. Add cinnamon, salt, and pepper. Stir, cook for another 2 minutes, then remove from the heat. In a bowl mix the eggs, hazelnuts, cream and pepper, as well as the garlic mix. Whisk thoroughly before pouring into the pan that they cooked garlic. Spread the mixture, place everything into the oven, and bake to 425 F in 10 mins. Slice, divide into plates and serve with breakfast.

Nutrition: calories 251, fat 5, fiber 8, carbs 17, protein 7

Leeks and Eggs Mix

Ingredients for 4 servings:
- 3 leeks, sliced   8 eggs, whisked
- 1 tablespoon avocado oil
- ¼ cup almond milk
- Salt and black pepper to the taste
- ¼ teaspoon garlic powder
- 1 teaspoon sweet paprika
- 1 tablespoon cilantro, chopped

Instructions: (5 minutes preparation time, 15 minutes cooking time):

In a fry pan, heat the oil on medium temperature, add the garlic powder, leeks and the paprika. Stir and cook for 5 minutes. Add the eggs along together with milk, salt and pepper. Stir and cook for another 10 minutes Divide the eggs among plates, add the cilantro and serve.

Nutrition: calories 340, fat 12, fiber 3.2, carbs 8, protein 23

Baked Eggs with Sausage

Preparation time: 10 minutes

Cooking time: 40 minutes

Servings: 6

Ingredients:

- 1 pound sausage, chopped
- 1 leek, chopped
- 8 eggs, whisked
- ¼ cup coconut milk
- 6 asparagus stalks, chopped
- 1 tablespoon fresh dill, chopped
- Salt and ground black pepper, to taste
- ¼ teaspoon garlic powder

- 1 tablespoon coconut oil, melted

Directions:

Heat a pan over medium heat, add sausage pieces, and brown for a few minutes. Add leeks and asparagus. Stir, then cook for a couple of minutes. In a bowl make a mixture of eggs, salt, pepper, dill curry powder and coconut milk and whisk. Pour the mix into an oven dish coated using coconut oil. Put the sausage and other vegetables over the top, and mix. Put in oven at 325 F. Bake in the oven for about 40 minutes. Serve warm.

Nutrition: Calories – 397, Fat – 32, Fiber – 1, Carbs – 4, Protein – 23.1

Spicy Frittata

Preparation time: 10 minutes

Cooking time: 15 minutes

Servings: 4

Ingredients:
- 1 green bell pepper, chopped
- 2 Serrano peppers, chopped
- 4 eggs, whisked
- ½ teaspoon turmeric powder
- 1 small yellow onion, chopped
- A pinch of salt and black pepper
- 4 bacon slices, chopped
- 10 cherry tomatoes, halved

Directions:

In a bowl mix the bell pepper with Serrano peppers, eggs, onion, turmeric, salt, pepper, and bacon. Mix well before pouring into the pan. Add cherry tomatoes, place to the oven and roast at 390 degrees F in 15 mins. Slice, divide among plates and serve with breakfast.

Nutrition: calories 261, fat 4, fiber 7, carbs 16, protein 8

Broccoli and Eggs Salad

Ingredients for 4 servings:
- 1 pound broccoli florets, steamed
- 4 eggs, hard boiled, peeled and cut into wedges
- 2 spring onions, chopped

- ½ teaspoon chili powder
- 1 tablespoon olive oil
- 1 tablespoon lime juice
- Salt and black pepper to the taste

Instructions: (10 minutes preparation time, 0 minutes cooking time):

In a bowl mix the eggs with the broccoli along with the other ingredients, toss and serve for breakfast.

Nutrition: calories 250, fat 11.2, fiber 4, carbs 5.6, protein 6.20

Chorizo and Cauliflower Breakfast

Preparation time: 10 minutes

Cooking time: 45 minutes

Servings: 4

Ingredients:

- 1 pound chorizo, chopped
- 12 ounces canned green chilies, chopped
- 1 onion, peeled and chopped
- ½ teaspoon garlic powder
- Salt and ground black pepper, to taste
- 1 cauliflower head, separated into florets
- 4 eggs, whisked
- 2 tablespoons green onions, chopped

Directions:

Heat a pan over medium heat, add chorizo, onion, stir, and brown for a few minutes. Add green chilies, stir, cook for a few minutes, and take off heat. In a food processor, blend cauliflower with salt and pepper, and blend. Transfer the mixture to an egg bowl, then add eggs and salt garlic powder, pepper and chorizo, mix then transfer to a well-greased baking dish. Bake in the oven at 375 F for about 40 minutes. Allow the casserole to cool for a few minutes. Sprinkle on green onions on top, Slice, and serve.

Nutrition: Calories – 883, Fat – 52.8, Fiber – 26.7, Carbs – 68.2, Protein – 43.5

Asparagus Frittata

Preparation time: 10 minutes

Cooking time: 30 minutes

Servings: 4

Ingredients:

- 4 bacon slices, chopped
- 8 eggs, whisked
- 1 bunch asparagus, trimmed and chopped
- A pinch of salt and black pepper

Directions:

In a fry pan, heat to medium-high flame, add bacon stirring until cooked for five minutes. Add asparagus and salt and pepper, stir, and cook for an additional 5 minutes. Whisked eggs are added, spread onto the pan, place into the oven, and bake to 350 degrees F in 20 mins. Slice, divide among plates, and serve as breakfast.

Nutrition: calories 251, fat 6, fiber 8, carbs 16, protein 7

Zucchini Casserole

Ingredients for 4 servings:
- 1 pound zucchinis, roughly cubed
- 1 cup mozzarella, shredded
- 1 shallot, chopped
- 1 tablespoon avocado oil
- 1 cup cherry tomatoes, chopped
- 4 eggs, whisked
- 1 tablespoon cilantro, chopped
- Salt and black pepper to the taste
- ½ cup kalamata olives, pitted and sliced

Instructions: (10 minutes preparation time, 35 minutes cooking time):

Prepare a pan using the oil on medium temperature, add the zucchini and shallot in 3 minutes and let them cook. Add olives, tomatoes and salt and pepper Stir, cook for another 2 minutes. Add the eggs, seasoned with cheese and cilantro on top, then spread over the zucchinis, bake in the oven and bake at 350 temperatures F in 30 mins. Let the casserole cool before serving it in slices.

Nutrition: calories 135, fat 8.1, fiber 2.5, carbs 7.8, protein 9.5

Italian Spaghetti Casserole

Preparation time: 10 minutes
Cooking time: 55 minutes
Servings: 4

Ingredients:

- 4 tablespoons butter
- 1 spaghetti squash, halved
- Salt and ground black pepper, to taste
- ½ cup tomatoes, cored and chopped
- 2 garlic cloves, peeled and minced
- 1 cup onion, peeled and chopped
- ½ teaspoon Italian seasoning
- 3 ounces Italian salami, chopped
- ½ cup Kalamata olives, chopped
- 4 eggs
- ½ cup fresh parsley, chopped

Directions:

Put squash pieces on a baking sheet, sprinkle with pepper and salt, then spread 1 tablespoon butter on them, bake at 400 F, then cook for about 45 mins. In a fry pan, melt the rest of the butter over medium-low heat. Add onions, garlic, salt and pepper, stir, cook for about a few minutes. Add the tomatoes and salami. Stir, then cook for about 10 minutes. Mix in the olives and cook for a couple of minutes. Remove the squash pieces from baking, scrape the flesh with a fork before adding together with the salami mixture in the pan. Mix, create 4 holes in the mix Crack an egg into each, and sprinkle salt and pepper, then place the pan in oven at 400 F and bake until eggs are done. Sprinkle the parsley over and serve.

Nutrition: Calories – 220, Fat – 18.1, Fiber – 1.7, Carbs – 9.4, Protein – 7

Herbed Frittata

Preparation time: 10 minutes
Cooking time: 30 minutes
Servings: 4

Ingredients:

- 12 eggs, whisked
- 4 tomatoes, chopped
- 1 yellow onion, chopped
- 8 bacon slices, chopped
- 1 tablespoon oregano, chopped

- 1 tablespoon basil, chopped
- 1 tablespoon parsley, chopped
- A pinch of salt and black pepper

Directions:

In a fry pan, heat it up to medium-high heat. Add bacon stir and boil for about 5 mins. Add the onion, stir and cook for 2 to 3 minutes. Add tomatoes, salt, pepper and basil, parsley and oregano. Stir, cook for one minute. Whisked eggs add, mix then bake in a 350 degree F over 20 minutes. Slice, divide among plates and serve with breakfast.

Nutrition: calories 251, fat 3, fiber 7, carbs 17, protein 7

Creamy Walnuts Bowls

Ingredients for 2 servings:

- 1 teaspoon nutmeg, ground
- 1 and ½ cups walnuts
- 1 teaspoon stevia
- 1 teaspoon vanilla extract
- ¾ cup coconut cream

Instructions: (5 minutes preparation time, 10 minutes cooking time):

In a saucepan, heat it up to medium-high heat. Add the walnuts, nutmeg, as well as the other ingredients, mix and simmer for 10 minutes, then divide into bowls and serve.

Nutrition: calories 200, fat 12, fiber 4, carbs 8, protein 4.5

Veggie Frittata

Preparation time: 10 minutes
Cooking time: 35 minutes
Servings: 4

Ingredients:

- ½ pound bacon, chopped
- 1 carrot, chopped
- 1 yellow onion, chopped
- 5 ounces mushrooms, chopped
- 1 bunch asparagus, chopped
- 8 eggs, whisked
- A pinch of salt and black pepper
- ¼ cup basil, chopped

Directions:

Heat a pan over medium-high heat, add bacon, stir and cook for 5 minutes. Add mushrooms, onion and asparagus and carrots, stirring and cooking for an additional 5 minutes. Add eggs, salt, pepper and basil, mix in the pan, then spread it out then bake and bake to 350 degrees F for about 25 minutes. Slice the frittata and divide it into plates, and serve it for breakfast.

Nutrition: calories 288, fat 3, fiber 6, carbs 18, protein 7

Coconut Berries Bowls

Ingredients for 4 servings:
- 1 cup blackberries   1 cup strawberries
- 1 cup raspberries
- 1 tablespoon lime juice
- ¼ cup almonds, cubed
- 2 teaspoons coconut oil, melted

Instructions: (5 minutes preparation time, 0 minutes cooking time):

In a bowl, combine the strawberries with the blackberries and the rest of the ingredients, toss, divide into small bowls and serve for breakfast.

Nutrition: calories 200, fat 7.5, fiber 4, carbs 5.7, protein 8

Granola

Preparation time: 10 minutes
Cooking time: 0 minutes
Servings: 2

Ingredients:

- 2 tablespoons chocolate, chopped
- 7 strawberries, hulled, and chopped
- A splash of lemon juice
- 2 tablespoons pecans, chopped

Directions:

In a bowl combine the chocolate with pecans, strawberries, as well as lemon juice. Mix well,

and serve chilled.

Nutrition: Calories – 167, Fat – 13.2, Fiber – 2.7, Carbs – 11.5, Protein – 2.6

Delicious Pork Frittata

Preparation time: 10 minutes
Cooking time: 15 minutes
Servings: 3

Ingredients:
- 2 tablespoons jalapeno, chopped
- 2 tablespoons cilantro, chopped
- 6 eggs, whisked
- 1 cup pulled pork meat, cooked
- 2 shallots, chopped
- 1 teaspoon avocado oil
- A pinch of salt and black pepper

Directions:

Prepare a pan using the oil at medium-high. Add jalapeno and shallots, stir and cook for about 2 minutes. Add pork, salt, and pepper. Stir and cook for another 2 minutes. Add eggs, mix in the pan, then pour in the pan, then place into the oven to heat to 425 degrees F in 10 mins. Slice, divide into plates, sprinkle with cilantro on top, and serve.

Nutrition: calories 261, fat 6, fiber 8, carbs 17, protein 6

Chia Bowls

Ingredients for 2 servings:
- ¼ cup walnuts, chopped
- 1 and ½ cups almond milk
- 2 tablespoons chia seeds
- 1 tablespoon stevia
- 1 teaspoon vanilla extract

Instructions: (10 minutes preparation time, 0 minutes cooking time):

In a bowl mix the almond milk, Chia seeds and other ingredients. Mix well, then set the mix to rest for 10 minutes before serving as breakfast.

Nutrition: calories 200, fat 8.3, fiber 2, carbs 5, protein 4

Almond Cereal

Preparation time: 5 minutes
Cooking time: 0 minutes.
Servings: 2

Ingredients:

- 2 tablespoons almonds, chopped
- 2 tablespoons sunflower seeds, roasted
- ⅓ cup coconut milk
- 1 tablespoon chia seeds
- ⅓ cup water
- ½ cup blueberries

Directions:

In a bowl, mix chia seeds with coconut milk, and set aside for 5 minutes. In the food processor, mix one half of sunflower seeds with almonds, and blend to a smooth. Mix this with the chia seed mixture. Mix in water and stir. Serve with the rest of the blueberries, sunflower seeds and serve.

Nutrition: Calories – 181, Fat – 15.2, Fiber – 4, Carbs – 10.8, Protein – 3.7

Leeks Breakfast Mix

Preparation time: 10 minutes
Cooking time: 20 minutes
Servings: 6

Ingredients:
- 6 eggs, whisked
- 12 bacon slices, chopped
- 4 leeks, chopped
- 1 pound collard greens, chopped
- 1 pint cherry tomatoes, sliced
- A pinch of salt and black pepper

Directions:

Heat a pan over medium-high heat, add bacon, stir and cook for 2-3 minutes. Add leeks, collards greens tomatoes, salt and pepper. Stir and cook for two minutes more. Add whisked eggs, mix in the pan, then pour into the pan and cook for another 2 minutes and then place in the oven to heat to 350 degrees F in 12 mins. Divide the mix among plates and serve it for breakfast.

Nutrition: calories 312, fat 12, fiber 6, carbs 14, protein 17

Tomato and Avocado Salad

Ingredients for 4 servings:
- 2 cups cherry tomatoes, halved
- 2 avocados, pitted, peeled, and cut into wedges
- A pinch of salt and black pepper
- 1 tablespoon olive oil
- 1 cucumber, sliced
- ½ cup kalamata olives, pitted and halved
- 1 tablespoon lime juice

Instructions: (5 minutes preparation time, 0 minutes cooking time):

Within a bowl mix the avocados with the tomatoes and the other ingredients. Mix and serve as breakfast.

Nutrition: calories 400, fat 9.2, fiber 4, carbs 5.5, protein 13.2

Nutty Breakfast Bowl

Preparation time: 5 minutes
Cooking time: 0 minutes
Servings: 1

Ingredients:

- 1 teaspoon pecans, chopped
- ½ cup coconut milk
- 1 teaspoon walnuts, chopped
- 1 teaspoon pistachios, chopped
- 1 teaspoon almonds, chopped
- 1 teaspoon pine nuts, raw
- 1 teaspoon sunflower seeds, raw
- 1 teaspoon stevia
- 2 teaspoons raspberries

Directions:

Mix milk in a bowl and honey, and stir. Add walnuts, pecans, almonds, pistachios and almonds, pine nuts, and sunflower seeds. Stir well, garnish with raspberries and serve.

Nutrition: Calories – 435, Fat – 44.2, Fiber – 5.2, Carbs – 10.8, Protein – 6.2

Spinach Pesto Eggs Mix

Preparation time: 10 minutes

Cooking time: 15 minutes

Servings: 4

Ingredients:

- 8 eggs, whisked
- 7 bacon slices, chopped
- 1 scallion, chopped
- 2 mushrooms, chopped
- 3 tablespoons spinach pesto
- 3 tablespoons olive oil
- A pinch of salt and white pepper

Directions:

In a pan, heat the oil on medium-high heat and add scallions. Stir until they are cooked for two minutes. Add bacon and stir, then cook for another 3 minutes. Add the mushrooms, salt and pepper mix and cook for one minute. Put the ingredients in a bowl and mix the eggs and pesto, stir thoroughly, pour over the mixture into the saucepan, stir with spread, place to the oven and bake at 400 F over 10 minutes. Divide the mix among plates and serve with breakfast.

Nutrition: calories 290, fat 12, fiber 5, carbs 17, protein 11

Salmon Cakes

Ingredients for 4 servings:

- 1 pound salmon fillets, boneless, skinless and minced
- 1 egg, whisked
- 2 spring onions, chopped
- 1 tablespoon cilantro, chopped
- 2 tablespoons almond flour
- A pinch of salt and black pepper
- 2 tablespoons olive oil

Instructions: (5 minutes preparation time, 10 minutes cooking time):

In a bowl mix the salmon with the egg, and all the other ingredients, excluding the oil. Stir well before shaping medium-sized cakes out of the mix. Prepare a pan using the oil on medium heat.

Add the salmon cakes and cook for 5 minutes each side, then divide them between plates and serve them for breakfast.

Nutrition: calories 249, fat 16.8, fiber 0.6, carbs 1.4, protein 24.3

Breakfast Bread

Preparation time: 10 minutes

Cooking time: 3 minutes

Servings: 4

Ingredients:

- ½ teaspoon baking powder
- ⅓ cup almond flour
- 1 egg, whisked
- A pinch of salt
- 2½ tablespoons coconut oil

Directions:

Make sure to grease a large microwave-safe mug with oil. In the bowl, mix egg with salt, flour oil, baking powder. Place the mix in a mug and microwave for three minutes on high. Allow the bread to cool before removing it from the mug, slice and serve.

Nutrition: Calories – 343, Fat – 38.5, Fiber – 0.4, Carbs – 0.8, Protein – 2.1

Shrimp and Eggs Mix

Preparation time: 10 minutes

Cooking time: 10 minutes

Servings: 4

Ingredients:

- 1 tablespoon olive oil
- 1 cup artichoke hearts, quartered
- ½ pounds shrimp, peeled and deveined
- 8 eggs
- 1/3 cup coconut cream
- A pinch of salt and black pepper
- 10 cherry tomatoes, halved

Directions:

Prepare a pan using the oil at medium-high Add shrimp and artichokes mix and cook until 3 mins. Within a bowl mix the eggs, cream, salt and pepper. Mix well, then put in the skillet, cover with it out, add cherry tomatoes and halves then cover the pan. Simmer for 10 minutes. Divide the mixture between plates and serve it for breakfast.

Nutrition: calories 261, fat 4, fiber 7, carbs 16, protein 8

Kale Frittata

Ingredients for 4 servings:
- 8 eggs, whisked
- 2 shallots, chopped
- 1 tablespoon avocado oil
- 1 cup kale, torn
- Salt and black pepper to the taste
- ¼ cup mozzarella, shredded
- 2 tablespoons chives, chopped

Instructions: (10 minutes preparation time, 30 minutes cooking time):

In a pan, heat the oil at medium-low temperature, add the shallots, stir to cook, stirring for five minutes. Add the kale, stir and cook for another 4 minutes. Add the eggs mixed with the mozzarella, spread into the pan, sprinkle the chives on top and bake at 390 F for 20 minutes. Divide the frittata between plates and serve.

Nutrition: calories 140, fat 6.7, fiber 1, carbs 4.3, protein 10

Breakfast Muffins

Preparation time: 10 minutes

Cooking time: 30 minutes

Servings: 4

Ingredients:

- ½ cup almond milk
- 6 eggs
- 1 tablespoon coconut oil
- Salt and ground black pepper, to taste
- ¼ cup kale, chopped
- 8 prosciutto slices
- ¼ cup fresh chives, chopped

Directions:

In a bowl make a mixture of eggs, salt, pepper, milk, kale, and chives. Grease a muffin tray using coconut oil, and cover with prosciutto slices and pour the egg mixture on top into the tray, bake in the oven baking at 350 F, for about 30 minutes. Transfer the muffins onto a plate and serve.

Nutrition: Calories – 257, Fat – 19.5, Fiber – 0.8, Carbs – 3.4, Protein – 18.1

Porridge

Preparation time: 10 minutes

Cooking time: 5 minutes

Servings: 2

Ingredients:

- ½ cup almonds, ground
- ½ cup coconut cream
- 1 teaspoon stevia
- ¼ cup water
- ¼ teaspoon nutmeg, ground
- ¼ teaspoon cloves, ground
- 1 teaspoon cinnamon powder

Directions:

In a small saucepan, heat with the water at a medium-low heat. Add the almonds, cream, stevia, cloves, nutmeg and cinnamon mix well, cook for five minutes. Serve in bowls.

Nutrition: calories 231, fat 4, fiber 8, carbs 16, protein 10

Spinach and Cauliflower Pan

Ingredients for 4 servings:
- 1 pound cauliflower florets
- 1 cup baby spinach
- 2 shallots, chopped   1 tablespoon olive oil
- 1 tablespoon balsamic vinegar
- 1 tablespoon parsley, chopped
- ½ cup walnuts, roughly chopped
- Salt and black pepper to the taste

Instructions: (10 minutes preparation time, 18 minutes cooking time):

Prepare a pan using the oil on medium heat. Add the shallots, stir then cook 3 mins. Add the cauliflower, and the other ingredients, toss and cook on medium temperatures for another 15 minutes Divide into bowls and serve as breakfast.

Nutrition: calories 140, fat 9.3, fiber 3, carbs 4, protein 8

Vegetable Breakfast Bread

Preparation time: 10 minutes
Cooking time: 25 minutes
Servings: 7

Ingredients:

- 1 cauliflower head, separated into florets
- ½ cup fresh parsley, chopped
- 1 cup spinach, torn
- 1 onion, peeled and chopped
- 1 tablespoon coconut oil
- ½ cup pecans, ground
- 3 eggs
- 2 garlic cloves, peeled and minced
- Salt and ground black pepper, to taste

Directions:

In a food processor, combine the cauliflower florets, adding salt and pepper and process until smooth. In a fry pan, heat oil over medium-high temperature, add the onions, cauliflower, garlic, along with salt, and some pepper stir and cook for about 10 minutes. In a bowl mixing eggs with salt pepper, parsley, nuts, spinach and stir. Mix in the cauliflower and mix well. Form the mixture into shapes and place on baking sheets, turn oven on to 350 F then bake 15 mins. Serve warm.

Nutrition: Calories – 105, Fat – 8.2, Fiber – 2.2, Carbs – 5.2, Protein – 4.2

Easy 5minute N-oatmeal

Ingredients for 1 serving:
- 1 teaspoon cinnamon
- 2 tablespoons approved sweetener
- 2 tablespoons grass-fed butter or coconut oil
- 2 cups coconut milk, unsweetened

- 1/4 cup flaxseed meal
- 1/4 cup coconut flour

Instructions (5 minutes preparation time, 5 minutes cooking time):

Add in milk, sweetener, flaxseed meal, coconut flour and cinnamon in a saucepan. Combine all the components together and place the pot at a medium temperature while stirring until the mixture becomes thicker. Remove from the heat and let it cool down until it is comfortable to manage. Add in butter and combine well Garnish the dish with low carb berries and almond flakes.

Calories 274, Carbs: 14 g, Protein: 5.4g, Fat: 21

Salad And Soups

Chicken Enchilada Soup

Preparation time: 20 minutes

Cooking time: 3 hours 10 minutes

Gross time: 3 hours 30 minutes

Serves: 2 to 4 people

Recipe Ingredients:

- 2 tsp. of olive oil (10 ml)
- 1 red onion (110 g), peeled and finely chopped
- 2 tsp. of cumin powder (4 g)
- 1 tsp. of cayenne pepper (2 g)
- 2 cloves of garlic (6 g), peeled and finely chopped
- 4 chicken breasts (800 g), skinless and deboned
- 2 tsp. of dried oregano (2 g)
- 3 ½ cups of chicken broth (840 ml)
- ¾ can of diced tomatoes (300 g)
- 1 yellow bell pepper (120 g), chopped
- Salt and pepper to taste
- 2 slices tomato (45 g), halved to garnish
- 1 large avocado (200 g), diced to garnish
- Cilantro, finely chopped to garnish
- ½ red chili pepper (7 g), seeds removed and finely chopped to garnish

Cooking Instructions:

Chop the onion in pieces and save 2 tablespoons of it to use as garnish. Cook the onions in a pan with olive oil until they are soft and caramelized. About halfway through the cooking, you can add cayenne pepper, cumin and garlic. Add the chicken, onions and oregano to the cooker. Add the broth of the chicken and tomatoes. Cover and cook at least 2.5 hours. Add the bell peppers and cook for an additional 30 minutes. Shred the chicken. Add salt and pepper to the chicken. If you wish sprinkle with a tiny slice of avocado, tomato or red chili, cilantro and onions. Serve warm.

Feta & Sun-Dried Tomato Salad

Ingredients for 2 servings

- 5 sun-dried tomatoes in oil, sliced
- 3 oz bacon slices, chopped
- 4 basil leaves
- 1 cup feta cheese, crumbled
- 2 tsp olive oil
- 1 tsp balsamic vinegar
- Salt to taste

Directions and Total Time: approx. 10 minutes

Cook bacon pieces in a skillet at medium-low heat until crisp and golden for about 5 minutes. Remove the bacon using a perforated spoon and place aside. Set the sun-dried tomato on a plate for serving. Sprinkle feta cheese on top and then top by basil leaves. Sprinkle bacon crispy on top, drizzle olive oil, and then sprinkle with salt and vinegar.

Per serving: Cal 426; Net Carbs 5.5g; Fat 38g; Protein 17g

Chicken and Cabbage Stew

Preparation time: 10 minutes

Cooking time: 1 hour

Gross time: 1 hour 10 minute

Serves: 2 to 4 people

Recipe Ingredients:

- 3 tbsp. (45 ml) of coconut oil, to cook with
- 2 chicken breasts, diced
- 4 slices bacon, diced
- ½ onion, diced
- ½ cabbage, sliced
- 3 cups (720 ml) of water or chicken broth
- Salt and pepper, to taste

Cooking Instructions:

Sauce the bacon, chicken and onions in coconut oil till the chicken has cooked. Add in the cabbage and water and bring to the boil. Cook for approximately 1 hour on low heat, with the lid on. Add salt and pepper according to your preference. Serve immediately and enjoy!

Cobb Salad with Roquefort Dressing

Ingredients for 4 servings

- ½ cup Roquefort cheese, crumbled
- ½ cup whipping cream
- ¼ cup buttermilk
- ½ cup mayonnaise
- 1 tbsp Worcestershire sauce
- 1 tbsp chives, chopped
- 3 eggs, hard-boiled, chopped
- 1 chicken breast
- 4 oz bacon, cooked, crumbled
- 1 cup endive, chopped
- ½ romaine lettuce, chopped
- 1 cup watercress
- 1 avocado, pitted and diced
- 1 large tomato, chopped
- ½ cup feta cheese, crumbled
- Salt and black pepper to taste

Directions and Total Time: approx. 20 minutes

Within a bowl mix buttermilk, whipping cream, mayonnaise, Worcestershire sauce. Add the Roquefort cheese and salt, pepper and chives. Store in the refrigerator. Preheat the grill pan over high heat. Sprinkle it with salt and black pepper. Grill for three minutes on each side. Transfer the chicken to a plate, cool for 3 minutes and cut into bite-sized chunks. Place the endive, lettuce and watercress in a salad bowl. Add the avocado, tomatoes, bacon, eggs and chicken. Spread the feta cheese on the salad and drizzle it in the cheese sauce.

Per serving: Cal 627; Net Carbs 8g; Fat 48g; Protein 32g

Chicken "Ramen" Soup

Preparation time: 10 minutes

Cooking time: 10 minutes

Gross time: 20 minutes

Serves: 1 to 3 people

Recipe Ingredients:

- 1 chicken breast, sliced
- 4 cups (960 ml) of chicken broth (or chicken bone broth)
- 2 eggs
- 1 zucchini, made into noodles
- 1 tbsp. of ginger, minced
- 2 cloves of garlic, peeled and minced
- 2 tbsp. (30 ml) of gluten-free tamari sauce or coconut aminos
- 3 tbsp. (45 ml) avocado oil, to cook with

Cooking Instructions:

Pan-fry the chicken in avocado oil, in the large fry pan, until the chicken is cooked golden. Hard boil 2 eggs, then cut them into half. In an enormous pot and cook along with the garlic, ginger and tamari sauce. Then add the zucchini noodles. Cook for about 2 to 3 minutes to soften the noodles. Divide the broth into two bowls and top with boiling eggs and chicken breast pieces. Sprinkle with Tamari or hot sauce according to taste. Serve immediately and enjoy!

Pesto Caprese Salad with Tuna

Ingredients for 2 servings

- 4 oz canned tuna chunks in water, drained
- 1 tomato, sliced
- 1 ball fresh mozzarella, sliced
- 4 basil leaves
- ½ cup pine nuts
- ½ cup Parmesan, grated
- ½ cup extra virgin olive oil
- ½ lemon, juiced

Directions and Total Time: approx. 10 minutes

In a food processor, combine to blend the leaves of basil, the pine nuts, Parmesan cheese and extra-virgin olive oil to blend them until they are smooth. Mix in the juice of a lemon. Place the slices of tomato and cheese on a plate for serving. Sprinkle the tuna chunks and pesto on top, and serve.

Per serving: Cal 364; Net Carbs 1g; Fat 31g; Protein 21g

Chicken Noodle Soup

Preparation time: 15 minutes

Cooking time: 15 minutes

Gross time: 30 minutes

Serves: 2 to 4 people

Recipe Ingredients:

- 3 cups of chicken broth

- 1 chicken breast, chopped into small pieces
- 2 tbsp. of avocado oil
- 1 stalk of celery, chopped
- 1 green onion, chopped
- ¼ cup of cilantro, finely chopped
- 1 zucchini, peeled
- Salt to taste.

Cooking Instructions:

Slice the breast of the chicken. Add the avocado oil into a saucepan and Saute the diced chicken in there until cooked. Add chicken broth to same pan and allow it to simmer. Chop the celery, and then add it to the pan. Chop the green onion, and mix it into the pot. Chop the cilantro, and set it aside for a while. Add the zucchini noodles and the fresh cilantro in the pan. Cook for a few minutes. Add salt according to your preference and serve it immediately.

Sausage & Pesto Salad with Cheese

Ingredients for 2 servings

- ½ cup mixed cherry tomatoes, cut in half
- ½ lb pork sausage links, sliced
- 1 cups mixed lettuce greens
- ¼ cup radicchio, sliced
- 1 tbsp olive oil
- ¼ lb feta cheese, cubed
- ½ tbsp lemon juice
- ¼ cup basil pesto
- 6 black olives, pitted, halved
- Salt and black pepper to taste
- 1 tbsp Parmesan shavings

Directions and Total Time: approx. 10 minutes

Cook the sausages in warm olive oil over medium heat for 5-6 minutes, stirring often. Within a bowl of salad mix the mixed lettuce leaves, radicchio and pesto, feta cheese, black olives, cherry tomatoes and lemon juice, then mix thoroughly to make sure that everything is covered. Sprinkle with salt and black pepper, then mix in the sausages. Sprinkle on Parmesan shavings before serving.

Per serving: Cal 611; Net Carbs 7.5g; Fat 48g; Protein 31g

Asian Miso Soup Topped with Shrimp

Preparation time: 5 minutes

Cooking time: 5 minutes

Gross time: 10 minutes

Serves: 1 to 3 people

Recipe Ingredients:

- 2 (3 ounces or 85 g) packs of shirataki noodles, drained
- 3 cups of chicken broth (600 ml) or bone broth
- 1 tbsp. of tahini sauce (15 ml)
- 1 tbsp. of gluten-free tamari sauce or coconut aminos (15 ml)
- ½ pound of shrimp (225 g), peeled
- 1 tsp. of sesame oil (5 ml)
- 2 tbsp. of lemon juice (30 ml)
- 2 green onions (10 g), sliced at an angle
- 1 cup of spinach (30 g), thinly sliced
- Dash of hot sauce (optional)

Cooking Instructions:

Rinse the shirataki noodles very well, as per the packet instructions to eliminate the smell. It is also helpful to boil it a little and then wash it off. Remove it from the water and place it aside. In the meantime, heat the broth and add the tahini sauce and Tamari sauce. When the broth is steaming hot add the shrimp, sesame oil and lemon juice. Continue to cook until you're certain that the shrimp are cooked. Then, add the rinsed noodles to the broth alongside the green onion as well as thinly cut spinach. Warm to your liking. Divide into 2 bowls and serve right away with a splash or hot sauce.

Smoked Salmon, Bacon & Egg Salad

Ingredients for 4 servings

- 2 eggs
- 1 head romaine lettuce, torn
- 4 oz smoked salmon, chopped
- 3 slices bacon
- 4 cherry tomatoes, halved
- Salt and black pepper to taste
- Dressing: ½ cup mayonnaise
- ½ tsp garlic puree
- 1 tbsp lemon juice
- 1 tsp tabasco sauce

Directions and Total Time: approx. 20 minutes

In a bowl, mix well the dressing ingredients and set aside. Bring a pot of salted water to a boil. Pour each egg out of a tiny bowl, then slowly slide it into the water. Poach for a couple of minutes. Remove using a spoon that has holes and transfer to an absorbent paper towel to dry, then place on a plate. Place it in a pan at medium-high heat, and cook until crispy and browned for about 6 minutes, rotating once. Remove, allow cooling, and chop into small pieces. Combine the salad and bacon, smoked salmon and the dressing into a bowl. Divide the salad into plates, then top it with two eggs, and serve right away or chilled.

Per serving: Cal 321; Net Carbs 5.4g; Fat 24g; Protein 15g

Salmon Stew

Preparation time: 5 minutes

Cooking time: 20 minutes

Gross time: 25 minutes

Serves: 2 to 4 people

Recipe Ingredients:
- 32 ounces (or 1 liter) of chicken broth
- 3 (6 to 8ounces) of salmon filets
- 1 cup of parsley, chopped
- 3 cups of Swiss chard, roughly chopped
- 2 Italian squash, chopped
- 1 clove of garlic, crushed
- Juice from ½ a lemon
- Salt and pepper to taste
- 2 eggs

Cooking Instructions:

Pour the broth of chicken into a pan and begin making it hot. As the broth heats, chop the veggies and add them with the garlic that has been crushed to the pot. Then, chop the salmon into chunks or strips and add them to the pot. Include your lemon juice. Cook for 10 minutes at a moderate temperature. Crack two eggs in the pan, and stir it around (make sure you smash egg yolks). Add pepper and salt to taste. Serve right away and Enjoy!

Classic Egg Salad with Olives

Ingredients for 2 servings
- 4 eggs
- ¼ cup mayonnaise
- ½ tsp sriracha sauce
- ½ tbsp mustard
- ¼ cup scallions
- ¼ stalk celery, minced
- Salt and black pepper to taste
- 1 head romaine lettuce, torn
- ¼ tsp fresh lime juice
- 10 black olives

Directions and Total Time: approx. 15 minutes

Boil eggs in salted water on moderate heat for about 10 minutes. Once they have cooled, peel and cut them into bite-sized pieces. Place them in a salad bowl. Mix in the other ingredients, except for the scallions until everything is well blended. Sprinkle the scallions on top and then decorate with black olives before serving.

Per serving: Cal 442; Net Carbs 9g; Fat 32g; Protein 24g

Spinach & Brussels Sprout Salad

Ingredients for 2 servings
- 1 lb Brussels sprouts, halved
- 2 tbsp olive oil
- Salt and black pepper to taste
- 1 tbsp balsamic vinegar
- 2 tbsp extra virgin olive oil
- 1 cup baby spinach
- 1 tbsp Dijon mustard
- ½ cup hazelnuts

Directions and Total Time: approx. 35 minutes

Pre-heat oven up to 400 F. Drizzle the Brussels sprouts with olive oil, then sprinkle with salt and black pepper and then spread them out on a baking tray. Bake until they are tender, 20 minutes, turning them frequently. In a dry pan on medium-high temperature toast the hazelnuts for 2 minutes. Cool, and in a large stockpot warm olive oil on medium-high temperature. Add the garlic and the half-portion of chopped parsley. Reserve the rest for garnish. Mix in anchovies, tomatoes and vegetable broth, salt, pepper and red chili flakes. Turn the heat to high, and cook the dish to boiling. Reduce the heat to medium-low and cover the pot and cook for 20 minutes. Open the lid and add the Halibut. Cover it again and cook for another 8 to 10 minutes or until fish can easily break off. Remove from the heat and cut halibut into smaller pieces. Mix until evenly distributed the fish. Serve with the rest of the fresh parsley.

Per serving: Cal 511; Net Carbs 10g; Fat 43g; Protein 14g

Spicy Halibut Tomato Soup

Preparation time: 15 minutes

Cooking time: 50 minutes

Overall time: 1 hour 5 minutes

Serves: 6 to 8 people

Recipe Ingredients:

- 1 teaspoon of olive oil
- 2 cloves of garlic minced
- ¼ cup of parsley fresh, chopped
- 3 tomatoes diced, without peel
- 10 anchovies canned in oil, minced
- 6 cups of vegetable broth 3 bouillon cubes + 6 cups water
- 1 teaspoon of salt
- 1 teaspoon of black pepper
- 1 teaspoon of red chili flakes
- 1 lb. of halibut filets fresh, chopped

Cooking Instructions:

In a large pot, cook olive oil on medium-high temperature. Add the garlic and about half the chopped parsley. Reserve the rest to garnish. Mix in anchovies, tomatoes and vegetable broth salt, pepper and red chili chips. Then, increase the heat to high, and cook the dish to boiling. Reduce the heat to medium-low and cover the pot and cook for 20 minutes. Open the lid and add the Halibut. Replace the cover and cook for 8 to 10 minutes or until the fish falls and breaks apart. Remove from

the heat and cut halibut into pieces. Mix the ingredients to evenly distribute the fish. Serve with garnishes of the remaining fresh parsley.

Chicken Salad with Parmesan

Ingredients for 2 servings

- ½ lb chicken breasts, sliced
- ¼ cup lemon juice
- 2 garlic cloves, minced
- 2 tbsp olive oil
- 1 romaine lettuce, shredded
- 3 Parmesan crisps
- 2 tbsp Parmesan, grated Dressing
- 2 tbsp extra virgin olive oil
- 1 tbsp lemon juice
- Salt and black pepper to taste

Directions and Total Time: approx. 30 min + chilling time

In the Ziploc bag, add the chicken and lemon juice, as well as the garlic, and oil. Close in the bag and shake the bag to mix, then refrigerate for one hour. Heat the grill to medium and cook the chicken for around 2 minutes per side. Mix all the dressing ingredients together within a tiny bowl, and mix thoroughly. On a serving plate lay out salad leaves and Parmesan crisps. Sprinkle the dressing on top and mix for a good coating. Add your chicken, and Parmesan cheese. Serve.

Per serving: Cal 529; Net Carbs 5g; Fat 32g; Protein 34g

Creamy Leek & Salmon Soup

Preparation time: 5 minutes

Cooking time: 25 minutes

Gross time: 30 minutes

Serves: 2 to 4 people

Recipe Ingredients:

- 2 tablespoon of avocado oil
- 4 leeks, washed, trimmed and sliced into crescents
- 3 cloves of garlic, minced
- 6 cups of seafood OR chicken broth
- 2 teaspoons of dried thyme leaves

- 1 pounds of salmon, in bite size pieces
- 1 ¾ cup coconut milk
- Salt and pepper to taste (omit pepper for AIP)

Cooking Instructions:

Heat the avocado oil in a large saucepan or Dutch oven at a low-medium heat. Add the chopped garlic and leeks, cook until they are soft. Add the stock to the pot along with the thyme. Let it simmer for around 15 minutes. Season according to taste with salt and black pepper. Add the salmon and coconut milk back into the saucepan. Bring to a simmer, then cook until the salmon is translucent and tender. Serve immediately and enjoy!

Smoked Mackerel Lettuce Cups

Ingredients for 2 servings
- ½ head Iceberg lettuce, firm leaves removed for cups
- 4 oz smoked mackerel, flaked
- Salt and black pepper to taste
- 2 eggs
- 1 tomato, seeded, chopped
- 2 tbsp mayonnaise
- ¼ red onion, sliced
- 1 tsp lemon juice
- 1 tbsp chives, chopped

Directions and Total Time: approx. 20 minutes

Boil eggs in the small saucepan in salted water about 10 minutes. After that, wash the eggs under cold water, then peel them and chop them into pieces. Transfer them into a salad bowl. Add the smoked mackerel and tomatoes, and red onion and mix them all together using the help of a spoon. Combine the lemon juice, mayonnaise, salt and black pepper together in small bowls, and mix to combine. Place two lettuce leaves as cups and then divide the salad mix in between the leaves. Sprinkle with chives and serve.

Per serving: Cal 334; Net Carbs 8g; Fat 25g; Protein 26g

Thai Coconut Soup with Shrimp

Preparation time: 5 minutes

Cooking time: 30 minutes

Gross time: 35 minutes

Serve: 2 to 4 people

Recipe Ingredients:
- Broth:
- 4 cups of chicken broth
- 1.5 cups of full fat coconut milk
- 3 kaffir lime leaves or zest of 1 organic lime
- 1-inch of fresh lemongrass cut in slices or 1 teaspoon dried lemongrass
- 1 cup of fresh cilantro
- 3 or 4 dried Thai chilies or 1 jalapeno sliced
- 1-inch of piece of fresh galangal root
- Lemongrass, galangal and chilis together here)
- 1 tsp. of sea salt
- Soup:
- 100 grams of raw wild caught shrimp
- 1 tbsp. of coconut oil
- 30 grams of mushrooms (any kind) sliced.
- 30 grams red onion, sliced thinly
- 1 tbsp. of fish sauce or 1 anchovy finely smashed
- Juice of 1 lime
- 1 tbsp. of chopped cilantro to garnish

Cooking Instructions:

Combine all the ingredients into a sauce pan and cook at a low simmer for around 20 minutes. Pass the mixture by using a fine-mesh strainer and then pour back in the pot. Bring the broth back up to an ebullient simmer. Add the chicken or shrimp, and the anchovy or fish sauce. Add the diced onions and mushrooms. Allow to simmer for 10 minutes or until the meat is cooked. Add lime juice, to serve the dish in bowls, with the chopped cilantro for garnish.

Kale & Broccoli Slaw with Bacon & Parmesan

Ingredients for 2 servings

- 2 tbsp olive oil
- 1 cup broccoli slaw
- 1 cup kale slaw
- 2 slices bacon, chopped
- 2 tbsp Parmesan, grated
- 1 tsp celery seeds
- 1 ½ tbsp apple cider vinegar
- Salt and black pepper to taste

Directions and Total Time: approx. 10 minutes

Cook your bacon on a pan over medium-high heat until crisp in approximately 5 minutes. Place the bacon aside to cool. In a bowl for salad, mix the vinegar, olive oil as well as salt and pepper. Add the broccoli, kale and celery seeds. Mix thoroughly. Sprinkle bacon and parmesan to serve.

Per serving: Cal 305; Net Carbs 3.7g; Fat 29g; Protein 7g

Cheesy Zucchini Soup

Preparation time: 10 minutes

Cooking time: 20 minutes

Serves: 2 to 4 people

Recipe Ingredients:

- 2 tbsp. (30 ml) of coconut oil
- 1 medium onion (110 g), peeled and chopped
- 3 zucchinis (360 g), cut into chunks
- 2 cups (480 ml) of bone broth
- 1 tbsp. (8 g) of nutritional yeast
- Dash of freshly ground black pepper
- 1 tbsp. (15 ml) of coconut cream, for garnish
- 1 tbsp. of parsley, chopped, for garnish

Cooking Instructions:

On medium heat, Melt the coconut oil inside a big pot. Add the onions and cook until tender. Add the zucchinis as well as bone broth. Reduce to the simmer. Cover the pan partially with a lid, and let it cook for about 15 minutes or until all the zucchinis are fully cooked. They should easily slide off a fork once you pierce them. Mix in the nutritional yeast before removing the pan from the stove. Use a hand blender, or food processor crush the mixture into the consistency of a fine soup. Sprinkle with freshly crushed black pepper. Serve with a beautiful sprinkle of coconut cream, chopped parsley and a drizzle.

Turkey Bacon & Turnip Salad

Ingredients for 4 servings

- 2 turnips, cut into wedges
- 2 tsp olive oil
- 1/3 cup black olives, sliced
- 1 cup baby spinach
- 6 radishes, sliced
- 3 oz turkey bacon, sliced
- 4 tbsp buttermilk
- 2 tsp mustard seeds
- 1 tsp Dijon mustard
- 1 tbsp red wine vinegar
- Salt and black pepper to taste
- 1 tbsp chives, chopped

Directions and Total Time: approx. 40 minutes

Fry the turkey bacon in a skillet over medium heat until crispy, about 5 minutes. Put aside and then chop it into pieces. Place a baking sheet on top of parchment paper. Toss them with pepper and then drizzle with olive oil and bake to bake for about 25 minutes, at 390 F and turning halfway through. Allow to cool. Place the baby spinach in the base of a salad plate and cover with bacon, radishes, and turnips. Blend the buttermilk with mustard seeds, vinegar, mustard and salt. Sprinkle the dressing on the salad. Mix well, then sprinkle with olives and chives. Serve.

Per serving: Cal 135; Net Carbs 6g; Fat 10g; Protein 6g

Cabbage Soup

Preparation time: 15 minutes

Cooking time: 45 minutes

Gross time: 60 minutes

Serves: 2 to 4 people

Recipe Ingredients:

- 3 tbsp. (45 ml) of coconut oil, to cook with
- 1 small cabbage (green or purple), chopped
- 1 carrot, diced
- 3 stalks of celery, chopped
- ½ onion, chopped
- 1 tomato, diced
- 6 cups (1.5 l) of bone broth (or vegetable broth if vegan or vegetarian)
- 2 cloves of garlic, minced
- 2 tbsp. of parsley, chopped
- Salt and pepper, to taste

Cooking Instructions: Pour coconut oil into an enormous pot and then heat the pot. Saute the carrot, cabbage as well as celery and onions in coconut oil till the vegetables have slightly cooked. Add the diced tomatoes and bone broth into the pot and bring to a boil. Then let it simmer for 30 minutes, or until the cabbage is soft. Include the garlic, parsley, salt and pepper, according to the taste. Cook for 5 minutes, then serve.

Fiery Shrimp Cocktail Salad

Ingredients for 4 servings
- 2 tbsp olive oil
- ½ head Romaine lettuce, torn
- 1 cucumber, cut into ribbons
- ½ lb shrimp, deveined
- 1 cup arugula
- ½ cup mayonnaise
- 2 tbsp Cholula hot sauce
- ½ tsp Worcestershire sauce
- Salt and chili pepper to season
- 1 tbsp lemon juice
- 1 lemon, cut into wedges
- 4 dill weed

Directions and Total Time: approx. 15 min + cooling time

Sprinkle the shrimp with salt as well as chili pepper. Warm the olive oil on moderate heat. Fry in 3 minutes each side until opaque and pink. Let the shrimp rest to cool. Mix the lemon juice, mayonnaise, hot sauce and Worcestershire sauce, mix until it is smooth and creamy in a bowl. Divide the cucumber and lettuce into four glass bowls. Top

with shrimp and drizzle the hot dressing over. Sprinkle arugula over top and garnish using lemon wedges as well as dill. Serve.

Per serving: Cal 241; Net Carbs 3.9g; Fat 18g; Protein 14g

Spring Soup with Poached Egg

Preparation time: 5 minutes

Cooking time: 15 minutes

Serves: 1 to 3 people

Recipe Ingredients:
- 2 eggs
- 32 ounces (1 quart) of chicken broth
- 1 head of romaine lettuce, chopped
- Salt to taste

Cooking Instructions:

Bring the chicken broth to a boil. Reduce the heat and cook the two eggs for five minutes (for slightly runny eggs). Take the eggs out and place each in the bowl. Mix the chopped romaine lettuce to the broth to cook for a couple of minutes until the lettuce is slightly soft. Ladle the broth along with the lettuce into bowls. Serve it immediately and enjoy!

Chicken, Avocado & Egg Bowls

Ingredients for 2 servings
- 1 chicken breast, cubed
- 1 tbsp avocado oil
- 2 eggs
- 2 cups green beans
- 1 avocado, sliced
- 2 tbsp olive oil
- 2 tbsp lemon juice
- 1 tsp Dijon mustard
- 1 tbsp mint, chopped
- Salt and black pepper to taste

Directions and Total Time: approx. 25 minutes

Blanch the beans in salted, boiling water over moderate heat for about 4-5 minutes till the beans turn crisp and bright green. Refresh with cold water, then remove. In the same pot of boiling water add the eggs and cook for about 10 minutes. Remove to an ice bath to cool. Peel and cut the avocados. Warm the avocado oil in a pan over medium heat. In the pan, cook chicken until around 4 minutes. Divide the green beans between two salad bowls. Add eggs, chicken with avocado slices. In a second bowl, whisk together the juice of the lemon olive oil, mustard, salt, and pepper and drizzle it over the salad. Sprinkle with fresh mint and serve.

Per serving: Cal 692; Net Carbs 6.9g; Fat 53g; Protein 40g

Mint Avocado Chilled Soup

Preparation time: 5 minutes

Cooking time: 5 minutes

Gross time: 10 minutes

Serves: 1 to 3 people

Recipe Ingredients:
- 1 medium ripe avocado
- 2 romaine lettuce leaves
- 1 cup (240 ml) coconut milk, chilled
- 1 tbsp. (15 ml) of lime juice
- 20 fresh mint leaves
- Salt to taste

Cooking Instructions:

Put all the ingredients in the blender and mix thoroughly. It should appear thick, but it should not be as dense as puree. Chill in fridge for about 5 to 10 minutes. Serve right away and enjoy!

Spinach Salad with Pancetta & Mustard

Ingredients for 2 servings
- 1 cup spinach
- 1 large avocado, sliced
- 1 spring onion, sliced
- 2 pancetta slices
- ½ lettuce head, shredded
- 1 hard-boiled egg, chopped Vinaigrette
- Salt to taste
- ¼ tsp garlic powder
- 3 tbsp olive oil
- 1 tsp Dijon mustard
- 1 tbsp white wine vinegar

Directions and Total Time: approx. 20 minutes

Chop the pancetta into pieces and fry in a skillet on moderate heat for five minutes or until crisp. Put the pancetta aside and let it cool. Mix the lettuce, spinach, egg, spring onion in the bowl. Whisk the vinaigrette components in a different bowl. Pour the dressing over and mix until well-combined. Serve with pancetta and avocado. Serve immediately

Per serving: Cal 467; Net Carbs 7g; Fat 42g; Protein 12g

Thai Beef and Broccoli Soup

Preparation time: 5 minutes

Cooking time: 40 minutes

Gross time: 45 minutes

Serves: 2 to 4 people

Recipe Ingredients:
- 2 tbsp. of avocado oil or fat of choice
- 1 onion, chopped
- 2 tbsp. of Thai green curry paste, adjust to taste
- 2-inch of knob ginger, minced
- 2 garlic cloves, minced
- 1 serrano pepper, minced
- 1 lb. of ground beef
- 3 tbsp. of coconut amino
- 2 tsp. of fish sauce
- ½ tsp. of salt
- ½ tsp. of black pepper
- 4 cups of beef bone broth or chicken stock
- 2 large stalks of broccoli, cut into florets
- 1 cup of full-fat canned coconut milk
- Cilantro, garnish

Cooking Instructions:
Add the oil and onions to a Dutch oven and cook for

10 minutes, or until the onions turn golden. In the meantime, add curry powder as well as garlic, ginger, and serrano pepper, and stir for about a minute. After that you should mix in the ground beef, fish sauce, coconut amino, salt and pepper, and cook until the meat is just browning. Add the broth and lower the heat to medium low. Close the lid, and cook for approximately 20 minutes. Mix the broccoli pieces along with coconut milk into the pot. Cover the pot and cook for an additional 10 minutes. Lift the lid off then increase temperatures to high, and simmer for 5 minutes. Serve with a sprinkle of cilantro.

Mediterranean Artichoke Salad

Ingredients for 4 servings
- 6 baby artichoke hearts, halved
- ½ lemon, juiced
- ½ red onion, sliced
- ¼ cup cherry peppers, halved
- ¼ cup pitted olives, sliced
- ¼ cup olive oil
- ¼ tsp lemon zest
- 2 tsp balsamic vinegar
- 1 tbsp chopped dill
- Salt and black pepper to taste
- 1 tbsp capers

Directions and Total Time: approx. 30 minutes

Bring a pot of salted water to a boil. Include the artichokes. Reduce the heat, and the artichokes simmer or until the artichokes are tender. Drain the artichokes and put them in the bowl to cool. Mix in the other ingredients, except for the olives. Toss thoroughly to mix. Add the olives on top and serve.

Per serving: Cal 204; Net Carbs 9g; Fat 15g; Protein 6g

Bacon Cheeseburger Soup

Preparation time: 10 minutes

Cooking time: 50 minutes

Gross time: 60 minutes

Serves: 3 to 5 people

Recipe Ingredients:
- 5 slices of bacon
- 12 ounces of ground beef (80/20)
- 2 tablespoons of butter
- 3 cups of beef broth
- ½ teaspoon of garlic powder
- ½ teaspoon onion powder
- 2 teaspoon of brown mustard
- 1 ½ teaspoon of kosher salt
- ½ teaspoon of black pepper
- ½ teaspoon of red pepper flakes
- 1 teaspoon of cumin
- 1 teaspoon of chili powder
- 2 ½ tablespoon of tomato paste
- 1 medium dill pickle, diced
- 1 cup of shredded cheddar cheese
- 3 ounces of cream cheese
- ½ cup of heavy cream

Cooking Instruction:

In a fry pan, cook bacon until crisp, then put it aside. Put the ground beef in the bacon fat, and cook until it is browned to one side. Then flip and cook until brown on the opposite side. Transfer the beef into an oven, then transfer into the middle. Add the butter and spices to the pan. Let the spices cook for 30 to 45 seconds. Pour beef broth and tomato paste, cheese, mustard and pickles into the pot and simmer for about a minute until the cheese is melted. Cover the pot and reduce to the lowest setting. Cook for 20-30 minutes. Switch off the stove, and end with heavy cream and bacon crumbles. Stir thoroughly and serve.

Arugula & Watercress Turkey

Salad Ingredients for 4 servings
- 1 tbsp xylitol
- 1 red onion, chopped
- 2 tbsp lime juice
- 3 tbsp olive oil
- 1 ¾ cups raspberries
- 1 tbsp Dijon mustard Salt and black pepper to taste
- 1 cup arugula

- 1 cup watercress
- ½ lb turkey breasts, boneless
- 4 oz goat cheese, crumbled
- ½ cup walnut halves

Directions and Total Time: approx. 25 minutes

Start by making the dressing. In a blender mix lime juice, xylitol, 1 cup raspberries, mustard, 1 cup of water, onions, olive oil and salt. Blend until it is smooth. Pour this dressing into the bowl and put it aside. Cook a pan on moderate heat. Grease it by spraying cooking oil. Coat the turkey with salt and black pepper and cut in half. Place the skin side down in the pan. Cook for 8 minutes before flipping over to the opposite side and cook in 5 mins. Arrange arugula and watercress on an arrangement of salad plates, then sprinkle with the rest of the raspberries, walnut halves, goat cheese. Cut the turkey into slices, place on top of the salad, then garnish with the raspberries dressing for serving.

Per serving: Cal 411; Net Carbs 7g; Fat 32g; Protein 24g

Bacon Cheeseburger Soup

Preparation time: 10 minutes

Cooking time: 50 minutes

Gross time: 60 minutes

Serves: 3 to 5 people

Recipe Ingredients:
- 5 slices of bacon
- 12 ounces of ground beef (80/20)
- 2 tablespoons of butter
- 3 cups of beef broth
- ½ teaspoon of garlic powder
- ½ teaspoon onion powder
- 2 teaspoon of brown mustard
- 1 ½ teaspoon of kosher salt
- ½ teaspoon of black pepper
- ½ teaspoon of red pepper flakes
- 1 teaspoon of cumin
- 1 teaspoon of chili powder
- 2 ½ tablespoon of tomato paste
- 1 medium dill pickle, diced

- 1 cup of shredded cheddar cheese
- 3 ounces of cream cheese
- ½ cup of heavy cream

Cooking Instruction:

In a skillet, cook bacon until crisp, then put it aside. Put the ground beef in the bacon fat, and cook until it is browned to one side. Then flip and brown the opposite side. Transfer the beef into the pot and then move away from the side. Add the butter and spices to the pan. Let the spices cook for 30 to 45 seconds. Add tomato paste, beef broth, mustard, cheese and pickles into the pot and cook for a couple of minutes until the cheese is melted. Cover the pot and cook on the heat to low. Cook for 20-30 minutes. Then turn off the stove and add heavy cream and bacon pieces. Mix well, and serve.

Spinach Salad with Goat Cheese & Nuts

Ingredients for 2 servings
- 2 cups spinach
- ½ cup pine nuts
- 1 cup hard goat cheese, grated
- 2 tbsp white wine vinegar
- 2 tbsp extra virgin olive oil
- Salt and black pepper to taste

Directions and Total Time: approx. 20 min + cooling time

Preheat oven to 390 F. Sprinkle the goat cheese grated in 2 circles, on top of two pieces. Place them in the oven to wait for 10 mins to bake. Take two bowls of the same size and place them upside-down and then carefully place the parchment paper over to create an appearance of a bowl. Allow to cool for about 15 minutes. Divide the spinach between the bowls add salt and pepper, then drizzle with olive oil. Add pine nuts on top to serve.

Per serving: Cal 540; Net Carbs 4.4g; Fat 52g; Protein 19g

Thai-Style Prawn Salad

Ingredients for 2 servings
- 2 cups watercress
- 1 green onion, sliced
- ½ lb prawns, cooked
- 1 avocado, sliced
- 1 Thai chili pepper, sliced
- 1 tomato, sliced
- 1 tbsp cilantro, chopped
- ¼ tsp sesame seeds
- 1 tbsp lemon juice
- 2 tsp liquid stevia
- ½ tsp fish sauce
- 1 tbsp sesame oil

Directions and Total Time: approx. 20 minutes

Within a bowl mix the sesame oil, stevia as well as fish sauce along with lemon juice. Add the prawns and toss in a coating. Keep covered in the refrigerator until 10 mins. Combine avocado, watercress, tomato Thai chili pepper, green onion, on a serving plate. Serve with prawns, as well as drizzle the marinade all over. Add sesame seeds and chopped cilantro and serve.

Per serving: Cal 340; Net Carbs 5.8g; Fat 25g; Protein 25g

Meatless Keto Club Salad

Time: 10 Minutes | Serves 1

Macros: Calories: 329.67 | Fats: 26.32g | Carbs: 4.83g | Protein: 16.82g

Ingredients
- 3 tbsp of sour cream
- 3 tbsp of mayonnaise
- 1 tsp milk
- 1/4 tsp garlic salt
- ½ tsp onion powder
- 2 tsp dried basil
- 2 tsp parsley
- 3 hard boiled eggs, sliced
- 4 ounces cheddar cheese, cubed
- 3 cups of shredded lettuce
- ½ cup of tomatoes

- 1 cup cucumber
- 2tsp of mustard

Preparation

Mix all the ingredients (minus eggs) in a small bowl. Place eggs (shells and the entire) in a large cooking pot. In the cooking pot, add water till the eggs are covered, and there is 1 inch of clearance (note that eggs won't be floating). Set the pan over the fire and set the flame to high. When the water is boiling it, set the timer for 10 minutes. Cut and then mash the eggs. Place the eggs, tomatoes, lettuce, cucumber, eggs and Dijon mustard onto a platter or in the bowl. Serve it over salad. Serve with cheese

Modern Greek Salad with Avocado

Ingredients for 2 servings
- 1 red bell pepper, roasted and sliced
- 2 tomatoes, sliced
- 1 avocado, sliced
- 6 kalamata olives
- ¼ lb feta cheese, sliced
- 1 tbsp vinegar
- 1 tbsp olive oil
- 1 tbsp parsley, chopped

Directions and Total Time: approx. 10 minutes

Place the tomatoes on a serving plate and then place the avocado slices on top. Put the bell peppers and olives on top of the avocado slices, and place feta pieces onto the platter. Sprinkle with vinegar and olive oil and sprinkle with chopped parsley to serve.

Per serving: Cal 411; Net Carbs 5.2g; Fat 35g; Protein 13g

Caprese Salad

Time: 40 Minutes | Serves 1

Macros: Calories: 190.75 | Fats: 63.49g | Carbs: 4.58g | Protein: 7.79g

Ingredients
- 5 cloves of minced garlic or garlic salt

- 4 cups of tomatoes that have been chopped
- 3 tbsp avocado oil
- 4 cups baby spinach
- 10 pieces mozzarella balls
- 1 tbsp pesto
- 1 tbsp brine, mozzarella brine
- ¼ cup basil

Preparation

Set the oven at 400 degrees/204 degree C. Place tomatoes and garlic on a baking tray lined with baking paper and then spread avocado oil in the middle. Roast for 30 minutes. Blend the cheese brine and pesto to make the dressing. Put the spinach, tomatoes and garlic that have been roasted in the bowl. Serve the bowl with mozzarella (break into pieces first) followed by the vegetable mix. Serve the dressing over it.

Seared Rump Steak Salad

Ingredients for 2 servings

- 1 cup green beans, steamed and sliced
- ½ lb rump steak
- 3 green onions, sliced
- 3 tomatoes, sliced
- 1 avocado, sliced
- 2 cups Romaine lettuce, torn
- 2 tsp yellow mustard
- Salt and black pepper to taste
- 3 tbsp extra virgin olive oil
- 1 tbsp balsamic vinegar

Directions and Total Time: approx. 20 minutes

In a bowl mix mustard with salt, black pepper and balsamic vinegar and extra-virgin olive oil. Set aside. Preheat a grill pan over high heat while you season the meat with salt and pepper. Place the steak into the pan and let it cook for 4 minutes each side. Transfer to a chopping board and allow to sit for four minutes before cutting. In a salad bowl add the green onions, tomatoes, green beans, steak slices, and lettuce. Sprinkle the dressing on top and mix well in a bowl to coat. Serve with avocado slices. Serve.

Per serving: Cal 611; Net Carbs 8.4g; Fat 45g;

Protein 33g

Taco Salad

Time:30 Minutes | Serves 4

Macros: Calories: 250 | Fats: 25g | Carbs: 2.35g | Protein: 15g

Ingredients

- 1 cup of ground beef
- 1 cup of water
- Chopped lettuce
- Chopped tomatoes
- 2 avocadoes
- 2 tbsp taco seasoning
- Shredded cheese of your choice

Preparation

Place the pan on the stove and cook it over moderate temperature. When the pan is hot and is smoking put the beef in it. Brown the meat in the pan, stirring as needed, when it's cooked, drain the grease and move on to the next step. Pour in the water and then add the taco seasoning by stirring thoroughly. After that, allow the mixture of meat and seasoning cook until cooked all the way through. Place the beef in the plate. Serve it on top of the lettuce which has been chopped as well as avocado, tomatoes, and cheese. Give it a few minutes to allow the cheese to melt prior to serving. If you'd like to, add some salt and pepper.

Cheesy Beef Salad

Ingredients for 4 servings

- ½ lb beef rump steak, cut into strips
- 1 tsp cumin
- 3 tbsp olive oil
- Salt and black pepper to taste
- 1 tbsp thyme
- 1 garlic clove, minced
- ½ cup ricotta, crumbled
- ½ cup pecans, toasted
- 2 cups baby spinach
- 1 ½ tbsp lemon juice
- ¼ cup fresh mint, chopped

Directions and Total Time: approx. 15 minutes

Preheat the grill to medium heat. Rub the beef with salt, 1 tbsp of olive oil, garlic, thyme, black pepper, and cumin. Put it on the barbecue and grill to cook 10 minutes, turning at least once. Sprinkle the pecans in a dry pan on moderate heat and cook for about 2 minutes, stirring frequently. Transfer the beef that has been grilled onto a cutting table allow to cool and cut into strips. In a bowl for salad, add baby spinach, mint, the remaining olive oil, salt, juice of a lemon, some ricotta and pecans. Toss thoroughly to make sure it is well coated. Add the beef slices.

Per serving: Cal 437; Net Carbs 4.2g; Fat 42g; Protein 16g

Avocado and Chicken Salad

Time:20Minutes | Serves 1

Macros: Calories: 550 | Fats: 38g | Carbs: 10g | Protein: 40g

Ingredients

- 1 cup chicken, already cooked and shredded ½ medium sized cucumber
- 1 avocado
- 4 small tomatoes (cherry tomatoes work well) 2 small onions
- 3 tsp lime or lemon juice or zest
- 3 tbsp olive oil
- Pepper
- Salt

Preparation

Make the vegetables ready by cutting the vegetables into pieces. Cut the avocado into slices. Discard the skin and the pit, as you won't need them. Add the lime or lemon juice or zest in an olive oil and mix them. Then, place the chicken in a dish on a plate, but don't cook it, as it must be cool. Add the vegetables over it. (Note that this is a good way to use up leftovers from the evening before). Add the juice and olive oil mixture on the chicken and veggies, and combine them. Sprinkle salt and spice according to your preference.

Pickled Pepper Salad with Grilled Steak

Ingredients for 2 servings

- ½ cup feta cheese, crumbled
- 1 lb skirt steak, sliced
- Salt and black pepper to taste
- 1 tsp olive oil
- 1 cup lettuce salad
- 1 cup arugula
- 3 pickled peppers, chopped
- 2 tbsp red wine vinegar

Directions and Total Time: approx. 15 minutes

Preheat grill to high heat. Sprinkle the steak slices with black pepper and salt and drizzle them with olive oil. Grill the steaks on both sides to your desired degree of doneness, which takes about 5 to 6 minutes. Transfer to the bowl, cover and let them rest while you prepare the salad. Mix the salad ingredients, including the lettuce, pickled peppers, arugula along with vinegar into a bowl for salad. Sprinkle the beef on top and sprinkle with the feta cheese.

Per serving: Cal 633; Net Carbs 7.7g; Fat 34g; Protein 72g

Egg Salad with Avocado

Time:20Minutes | Serves 4

Macros: Calories: 250 | Fats: 52.5g | Carbs: 2.53g | Protein: 8.65g

Ingredients

- 6 large eggs
- 3 tbsp of lemon or lime juice
- 3 avocados
- 1 small red onion
- 3 tsp dill
- Salt
- Pepper

Preparation

Place eggs (shells and the eggs in all) in a saucepan. Pour in water until the eggs are covered , and there's 1 inch of space (note that eggs won't flounder). Set the pan over the fire and set the flame up to high. Once the water has reached a boil, you can set a timer for 10 minutes. Let the eggs be cool prior to peeling. The pit and skin off of the avocados and then mash them. Cut the onion into smaller pieces. Cut the eggs into pieces. Mix the avocado, red onion, eggs and seasonings. Serve

Parma Ham & Egg Salad

Ingredients for 4 servings

- 8 eggs
- 1/3 cup mayonnaise
- 1 tbsp minced onion
- ½ tsp mustard
- 1 ½ tsp lime juice
- Salt and black pepper to taste
- 10 lettuce leaves
- 4 Parma ham slices

Directions and Total Time: approx. 20 minutes

Boil eggs for about 10-15 minutes inside a saucepan filled with salted water. Remove the eggs and run them in cold, icy water. Then, peel and chop. Transfer the chopped ham to the mixing bowl along with mayonnaise, black pepper, mustard, onion, lime juice and salt. Serve with salad leaves, ham slices and pieces to serve.

Per serving: Cal 273; Net Carbs 1.6g; Fat 23g; Protein 15g

Cauliflower Salad

Time: 10 Minutes | Serves 10

Macros: Calories: 211.12 | Fats: 19.6g | Carbs: 2.82g | Protein: 4.92g

Ingredients

- 1 medium head cauliflower, chopped
- 4 hard boiled eggs, chopped
- 1 cup mayonnaise
- ⅓ cup bacon bits
- 2 tbsp apple cider vinegar
- ¼ cup onions, chopped
- 1 tsp garlic, minced
- ¾ cup of chopped green onions
- 1 tsp sugar substitute

Preparation

Mix the eggs, mayonnaise, bacon bits, eggs and apple cider vinegar, garlic, onions, sugar substitute, and green onions in the bowl. Stir until the entire

bowl is thoroughly combined. Slowly mix through the cauliflower until it is thoroughly blended. Serve warm

Chicken Salad with Gorgonzola Cheese

Ingredients for 2 servings

- ½ cup gorgonzola cheese, crumbled
- 1 chicken breast, boneless, skinless, flattened
- Salt and black pepper to taste
- 1 tbsp garlic powder
- 2 tsp olive oil
- 1 cup arugula
- 1 tbsp red wine vinegar

Directions and Total Time: approx. 15 minutes

Sprinkle the meat with black pepper, salt and garlic powder. Heat half of the olive oil in a pan over medium heat and fry the chicken for 4 minutes on both sides or until golden brown. Transfer the chicken to an eating board and allow to cool completely before cutting. Mix the arugula in vinegar and olive oil. Divide the salads on plates. Place the chicken slices on top and top the top with grated gorgonzola.

Per serving: Cal 421; Net Carbs 3.5g; Fat 28g; Protein 39g

Spinach and Watercress Salad

Time: 10 Minutes | Serves 4

Macros: Calories: 203.75 | Fats: 18.59g | Carbs: 1.85g | Protein: 5.32g

Ingredients

- 2cups of watercress that have been cleaned, prepared, and ready to use
- 3 cups baby spinach, cleaned and stemmed
- 1 avocado that has been sliced
- ½ cup of the shredded cheese of your choice
- ¼ cup avocado oil
- Salt
- Pepper

- Lemon or lime juice

Preparation

Blend the oil with lime or lemon juices along with salt and the black pepper (if you'd like to add the latter) in the bowl to make the dressing. Place the watercress and the spinach in a bowl. Add an avocado in the middle. Pour the dressing over them. Sprinkle your cheese shredded on the top.

Cheddar & Turkey Meatball Salad

Ingredients for 4 servings
- 3 tbsp olive oil
- 1 tbsp lemon juice
- 1 lb ground turkey
- Salt and black pepper to taste
- 1 head romaine lettuce, torn
- 2 tomatoes, sliced
- ¼ red onion, sliced
- 3 oz yellow cheddar, shredded

Directions and Total Time: approx. 30 minutes

Combine the turkey ground together with black pepper and salt, and form into meatballs. Refrigerate for 10 minutes. Cook half of the olive oil on a skillet at medium-high temperature. Fry the meatballs in both sides for about 10 minutes, until they are cooked and brown inside. Transfer the meatballs to a wire rack to drain the oil. Mix the tomatoes, lettuce and red onions in a bowl for salad, add the olive oil and salt, lemon juice and pepper. Mix and place the meatballs to top. Sprinkle the cheese on top of the salad. Serve.

Per serving: Cal 382; Net Carbs 3.5g; Fat 27g; Protein 30g

Taco Soup

Time: 5 Hours | Serves 8

Macros: Calories: 398 | Fats: 29g | Carbs: 6.9g | Protein: 28.5g

Ingredients
- 1 package ground beef
- ½ tsp red pepper flakes
- 2 tbsp of chili powder
- 2 tsp cumin
- 3 tsp red pepper flakes
- ½ tsp oregano
- Salt
- Pepper
- 2 packages of cream cheese
- 2 cans diced tomatoes
- 1 can of green chilis that have been diced 2 containers beef broth
- ½ cup heavy whipping cream

Preparations

Brown the ground beef on the stovetop in a pan, stirring until every piece is cooked thoroughly. The grease should be drained (depending upon the fat content of the meat you use there is no need for this) and then transfer the beef in a slow cooker. Include the other ingredients including the seasonings. Finally, mix whipping cream and stewed beef into the slow cooker. The lid of the slow cooker should be on and then turn the temperature to high for 4 hours. Serve and relax

Warm Cauliflower Salad

Ingredients for 4 servings
- 1 cup roasted bell peppers, chopped
- 2 tbsp celery leaves, chopped
- 10 oz cauliflower florets
- 1 red onion, sliced
- ¼ cup extra-virgin olive oil
- 1 tbsp wine vinegar
- 1 tsp yellow mustard
- Salt and black pepper to taste
- ½ cup black olives, chopped
- ½ cup cashew nuts

Directions and Total Time: approx. 15 minutes

Cook the cauliflower with salted water inside a pan at medium-low heat for 5 minutes. Drain, then transfer to the salad bowl. Include roasted peppers, red onion, and olives. In a small bowl add salt, mustard, olive oil, vinegar, and black pepper. Sprinkle the mix over the vegetables. Serve with cashew nuts and celery. Serve.

Per serving: Cal 213; Net Carbs 7g; Fat 16g; Protein 5g

Oven Baked Pork Chops with Salad

Time: 45 Minutes | Serves 2

Macros: Calories: 325 | Fats: 15.25g | Carbs: 5.67g | Protein: 52.3g

Ingredients

- 2 boneless pork chops
- 1 tsp pepper
- 1 tsp salt
- 1 tbsp garlic salt
- 1 tbsp dried parsley
- 1 tbsp dried basil
- 2 cups of lettuce
- 2 cups of spinach
- Cherry tomatoes
- Olive oil as necessary

Preparations

Place the pork chops in a baking pan that will not stick. Sprinkle them all over with the spices - garlic salt and parsley, basil, salt, and pepper in the same order. Bake at 350°F/176° C until cooked to perfection, and the inside has reached a temperature of 165°F/73 degree C. Clean both spinach and lettuce. Break them up into tiny pieces, then mix them by hand, stopping once they're well mixed. Make the tomatoes ready by cutting off the stem, then cutting them into half. Place the tomatoes over the lettuce and spinach. Add a small amount of olive oil over the salad you've recently prepared. Place the chops of pork on a dish with the salad beside them.

Arugula & Roasted Pepper Salad

Ingredients for 4 servings

- 2 lb red bell peppers, deseeded and cut into wedges
- 1/3 cup arugula
- ½ cup Kalamata olives, pitted
- 3 tbsp chopped walnuts
- ½ tsp Swerve sugar
- 2 tbsp olive oil
- 1 tbsp mint leaves
- ½ tbsp balsamic vinegar
- ¼ cup crumbled goat cheese
- Toasted pine nuts for topping

- Salt and black pepper to taste

Directions and Total Time: approx. 30 minutes

Pre-heat oven up to 400 F. Place bell peppers into a roasting pan. Sprinkle with sugar, then drizzle with half the olive oil. Bake for about 20 mins or till lightly burned; allow to cool. Place arugula in the bowl of a salad and sprinkle with roasted bell peppers walnuts, mint, olives and drizzle it with olive oil. Sprinkle with pepper and salt. Mix and serve the dish with cheese from goat and pine nuts.

Per serving: Cal 229; Net Carbs 10g; Fat 16g; Protein 6g

Greek Zoodle Mason Jar Salad

SERVES 2

Ingredients

- 2 tablespoons extra-virgin olive oil
- 2 tablespoons lemon juice
- 1 teaspoon dried oregano
- ¼ teaspoon sea salt
- ¼ teaspoon ground black pepper
- ½ cup cubed cooked chicken
- ¼ cup chopped peeled red onion
- ¼ cup chopped pitted Kalamata olives
- ¼ cup crumbled feta cheese
- 2 medium zucchini, spiralized

Mix lemon juice, olive oil, oregano and salt, pepper in one small bowl. Place 2 tablespoons of dressing into the bottom of two 1 quart wide-mouthed Mason Jars. Two layers of 1/4 cup of chicken, 2 tablespoons red onion, 2 tablespoons olives, 2 tablespoons of feta cheese and half of the zucchini noodles in each jar. Keep in the refrigerator for up to a week. Shake well prior to serving.

Smoked Salmon Salad

Ingredients for 2 servings

- 2 slices smoked salmon, chopped
- 1 tsp onion flakes
- 3 tbsp mayonnaise
- ½ Romaine lettuce, shredded

- 1 tbsp lime juice
- 1 tbsp extra virgin olive oil
- Sea salt to taste
- ½ avocado, sliced

Directions and Total Time: approx. 10 minutes

Mix ingredients like salmon, mayonnaise, lime juice, olive oil along with salt in a bowl and mix well. On a salad plate lay out the lettuce pieces and onion pieces. Spread the salmon mixture over and top with avocado slices.

Per serving: Cal 261; Net Carbs 2.2g; Fat 20g; Protein 10g

Cabbage Salad

Servings: 6

Cooking Time: 15 minutes

Ingredients

For Salad:

- 4 cups green cabbage, shredded
- ¼ onion, thinly sliced
- 1 teaspoon lime zest, grated freshly
- 3 tablespoons fresh cilantro, chopped

For Dressing:

- ¾ cup mayonnaise
- 2 teaspoons fresh lime juice
- 2 teaspoons chili sauce
- ½ teaspoon Erythritol
- 2 garlic cloves, minced

Directions:

To make the salad: in a bowl, mix the onions, cabbage, lime zest and cilantro. For dressing, combine all ingredients and mix until thoroughly combined in a second small bowl. Pour the dressing over the salad and gently stir in a well-coated dish. Cover and refrigerate until chilled prior to serving.

Nutrition Info (Per Serving): Calories: 196; Net Carbs: 2.3g; Carbohydrate: 3.6g; Fiber: 1.3g; Protein: 0.7g; Fat: 20.1g; Sugar: 1.7g; Sodium: 231mg

Greek Beef Meatball Salad

Ingredients for 4 servings

- 2 tbsp almond milk
- 1 lb ground beef
- 1 onion, grated
- ¼ cup pork rinds, crushed
- 1 egg, whisked
- 1 tbsp fresh parsley, chopped
- Salt and black pepper to taste
- 1 garlic clove, minced
- 1 tbsp fresh mint, chopped
- ½ tsp dried oregano
- 4 tbsp olive oil
- 1 cup cherry tomatoes, halved
- 1 Lebanese cucumber, sliced
- 1 cup butterhead lettuce, torn
- 1½ tbsp lemon juice
- 1 cup Greek yogurt

Directions and Total Time: approx. 20 minutes

In a mixing bowl mix almond milk, ground beef, salt, parsley, onion egg, black pepper, pork rinds, oregano and garlic. Form the mixture into balls. Warm the oil on a skillet on medium heat. Fry the meatballs in the oven for 8 to 10 minutes. Transfer them to a paper towel lined tray to drain. On a salad plate mix lettuce, cherry tomatoes and cucumber. Mix with the remaining oil and lime juice, black pepper and salt. Mix the yogurt with mint, then spread it on the salad. Top with meatballs, and serve.

Per serving: Cal 488; Net Carbs 6.3g; Fat 31g; Protein 42g

Buffalo Chicken Mason Jar Salad

SERVES 2

- 2 (4.5-ounce) cans cooked chicken breast
- ¼ cup The New Primal Medium Buffalo Dipping & Wing Sauce
- ¼ cup Tessemae's Organic Creamy Ranch Dressing
- 2 large hard-boiled eggs, roughly chopped
- 2 tablespoons minced seeded green bell pepper

- 2 tablespoons minced cucumber
- ¼ cup chopped black olives
- ½ cup chopped avocado
- 2 cups chopped romaine lettuce

Combine chicken breast and buffalo sauce in a medium bowl and toss to coat. Scoop 2 tablespoons of ranch dressing into the bottom of two 1-quart wide-mouthed Mason jars and layer equal parts chicken, one chopped egg, 1 tablespoon bell pepper, 1 tablespoon cucumber, 2 tablespoons black olives, 1/4 cup avocado, and 1 cup lettuce on top. Cover and keep within the fridge for up to one week. Once you're ready to eat it shake vigorously prior to serving.

Caprese Salad Stacks with Anchovies

Ingredients for 4 servings
- 4 anchovy fillets in oil
- 12 fresh mozzarella slices
- 4 red tomato slices
- 4 yellow tomato slices
- 1 cup basil pesto

Directions and Total Time: approx. 10 minutes

Pick up a serving tray and alternately place tomatoes or a slice of mozzarella, the yellow tomato slice, another slice of mozzarella and the red tomato slice and finally, a mozzarella slice on top. Repeat for 3 stacks the same way. Sprinkle pesto on top. Place anchovies on top and serve.

Per serving: Cal 292; Net Carbs 5g; Fat 20g; Protein 22g

Five-Minute Creamy Tomato Soup

SERVES 2
- 1 (15-ounce) can tomato sauce
- 1 (8-ounce) can tomato sauce
- 1 cup grass-fed half-and-half
- 1 ½ teaspoons golden monk fruit sweetener
- 1 teaspoon Italian seasoning
- ½ teaspoon dried basil

- ½ teaspoon dried parsley
- ½ teaspoon sea salt
- ¼ teaspoon ground black pepper
- ½ teaspoon Frank's RedHot Original Cayenne Pepper Sauce
- 3 tablespoons shredded Parmesan cheese

Mix all ingredients, except for Parmesan cheese in a medium-sized saucepan over medium-high temperature. Stir frequently until the mixture is heated to your liking, approximately 5 minutes. Add Parmesan cheese. Remove from the stove and serve.

Classic Greek Salad

Ingredients for 2 servings
- 3 tbsp extra virgin olive oil
- ½ lemon, juiced
- 2 tomatoes, sliced
- 2 Persian cucumbers, diced
- 1 red bell pepper, sliced
- 1 small red onion, chopped
- 10 Kalamata olives
- 4 oz feta cheese, cubed
- 1 tsp parsley, chopped
- Salt to taste

Directions and Total Time: approx. 10 minutes

Mix olive oil with lemon juice and salt in a bowl. In a salad bowl add cucumber, tomatoes, bell pepper, red onion and parsley. Toss in the dressing. Serve with olives and feta. Serve.

Per serving: Cal 288; Fat 28g; Net Carbs 7g; Protein 10g

BLT Chicken Mason Jar Salad

SERVES 2
- 4 tablespoons mayonnaise
- ½ teaspoon lemon juice
- 1 teaspoon minced green onion
- ⅛ teaspoon sea salt
- ⅛ teaspoon ground black pepper
- ½ cup chopped cooked no-sugar-added bacon
- 1 cup chopped cooked chicken

- 1 cup chopped Roma tomato
- ½ cup chopped avocado
- 2 cups chopped romaine lettuce

Mix mayonnaise with lemon juice, fresh green onions, salt and black pepper into a smaller bowl, and mix until smooth. Scoop 2 tablespoons dressing to the top of two wide-mouthed Mason Jars. Place 1/4 cup bacon, 1/2 cup chicken, 1/2 cup tomato, 1/4 cup avocado and 1 cup lettuce into each jar. Refrigerate for up to a week. Once you're ready to eat it shake vigorously, and serve.

Warm Mushroom & Pepper Salad

Ingredients for 4 servings
- 1 cup mixed mushrooms, chopped
- 2 tbsp sesame oil
- 2 yellow bell peppers, sliced
- 1 garlic clove, minced
- 2 tbsp tamarind sauce
- ½ tsp hot sauce
- 1 tsp sugar-free maple syrup
- ½ tsp ginger paste
- Chopped toasted pecans
- Sesame seeds to garnish
- Salt and black pepper to taste

Directions and Total Time: approx. 20 minutes

Heat Sesame Oil in the skillet at medium-low heat. Cook mushrooms and bell peppers for 8-10 mins. Sprinkle with salt and black pepper. In a bowl mix the garlic with the tamarind sauce, hot sauce, maple syrup along with ginger paste. Mix the ingredients into the vegetables and stir-fry for about two minutes. Sprinkle the salad in the sesame remaining oil and decorate with sesame seeds. Serve.

Per serving: Cal 291; Net Carbs 7.2g; Fat 27g; Protein 4g

Lemon Garlic Mason Jar Salad

SERVES 2

- 4 tablespoons Tessemae's Organic Lemon Garlic Dressing & Marinade
- ½ cup shredded cooked chicken breast
- ¼ cup chopped cucumber
- ½ cup chopped cherry tomatoes
- ¼ cup crumbled feta cheese
- ¼ cup chopped hard-boiled egg
- ¼ cup chopped avocado
- ⅛ cup chopped fresh cilantro
- 2 cups chopped romaine lettuce

Place 2 tablespoons of dressing in the bottom of two wide-mouthed Mason Jars. Take 1/4 cup chicken onto the top of the dressing. Layer each container with 2 tablespoons cucumber, 1/4 cup tomatoes, 2 tablespoons feta cheese, 2 tablespoons egg, 2 tablespoons avocado, 1 tablespoon cilantro and 1 cup of lettuce. Cover and place within the fridge for up to one week, or until you are ready to serve. When you are ready to eat shake vigorously, and serve it immediately.

Cauliflower-Watercress Salad

Ingredients for 4 servings
- 2 tbsp sesame oil
- 1 lemon, zested and juiced
- 10 oz cauliflower florets
- 12 green olives, chopped
- 8 sun-dried tomatoes, drained
- 3 tbsp chopped scallions A handful of toasted peanuts
- 3 tbsp chopped parsley
- ½ cup watercress
- Salt and black pepper to taste

Directions and Total Time: approx. 15 minutes

In a large pot, on medium heat, bring the water to boil. Set up a steamer basket and add the cauliflower. Soften for 8 minutes. Transfer the cauliflower into a salad bowl. Add tomatoes, olives and scallions, lemon juice and zest, Sesame oil, peanuts parsley, watercress and parsley. Sprinkle with salt and pepper. Mix with the spoon. Serve.

Per serving: Cal 198; Net Carbs 8.4g; Fat 10g; Protein 6g

Creamy Artichoke Soup

SERVES 6

- ¼ cup grass-fed butter
- ½ cup chopped celery
- 2 teaspoons minced garlic
- ¾ cup chopped peeled yellow onion
- ½ cup sliced white mushrooms
- 2 tablespoons arrowroot powder
- 2½ cups chicken bone broth
- 3 (12-ounce) jars quartered artichoke hearts, drained
- ½ teaspoon sea salt
- ½ teaspoon ground black pepper
- ½ teaspoon Italian seasoning
- ¼ teaspoon dried sage
- ⅛ teaspoon paprika
- 1 cup grass-fed half-and-half

In large stockpot on medium-high temperature. Add celery, garlic, mushrooms, and onion and cook until they soften approximately 5 minutes. Add the powder of arrowroot and stir it in to mix. Cook for another 5 minutes, while stirring regularly. Add the remaining ingredients, excluding half-and-half. Stir to mix. Reduce heat to low, and simmer for an hour. Mix in half and half, then heat until it is heated to your liking. Use an immersion blender to puree soup until smooth. Remove from heat and serve.

Shrimp Salad with Avocado

Ingredients for 4 servings

- 2 tomatoes, chopped
- ½ lb medium shrimp
- 3 tbsp olive oil
- 1 avocado, chopped
- 1 tbsp cilantro, chopped
- 1 lime, zested and juiced
- 1 head Iceberg lettuce, torn
- Salt and black pepper to taste

Directions and Total Time: approx. 20 minutes

Heat 1 tbsp olive oil in a skillet over medium heat and cook the shrimp until opaque, 8-10 minutes. Put the salad on a plate and then top it with tomatoes, shrimp, and avocado. Mix the olive oil

remaining and lime zest juice, salt and pepper in an ice-cold bowl. Serve the dressing on the salad and garnish with chopped cilantro before serving.

Per serving: Cal 249; Net Carbs 7.2g; Fat 18g; Protein 10g

Asian Cucumber Salad

Prep time: 10 mins., cook time: 15 min., total time: 25 min.

Serves: 4

Ingredients:

- $\frac{1}{5}$ packet shirataki noodles
- 3 tbsp. coconut oil
- $\frac{1}{2}$ medium spring onion
- $\frac{1}{4}$ tsp red pepper flakes
- 4 scoop whey protein
- $\frac{1}{4}$ large cucumber, thinly sliced
- 1 tbsp. Sesame oil
- $\frac{1}{4}$ tbsp. Rice vinegar
- 10 tsp. Sesame seeds
- $\frac{1}{2}$ tsp salt
- $\frac{1}{2}$ tsp freshly ground pepper

Instructions:

Dry and thoroughly rinse the Shirataki noodles. Cook the coconut oil on medium-high temperature. Add the noodles, then cover (to stop spilling) Cook for seven minutes. Add the other ingredients, mix and cook to a simmer for two additional minutes. If you're about to eat, spread thinly cut cucumber slices on a platter and then top with the noodles.

Nutritional information:

Calories 295, fat 19.6g, cholesterol 65mg, sodium 397mg, carbs. 7.8g, dietary fiber 1.2g, sugars 1.3g, protein 23.9g

Green Salad with Feta & Blueberries

Ingredients for 4 servings

- 2 cups broccoli slaw
- 2 cups baby spinach
- 2 tbsp poppy seeds
- 1/3 cup sunflower seeds
- 1/3 cup blueberries
- 2/3 cup chopped feta cheese
- 1/3 cup chopped walnuts
- 2 tbsp olive oil
- 1 tbsp white wine vinegar
- Salt and black pepper to taste

Directions and Total Time: approx. 10 minutes

In a bowl, whisk olive oil, vinegar, poppy seeds, salt, and pepper; set aside. In a salad bowl, combine the broccoli slaw, spinach, walnuts, sunflower seeds, blueberries, and feta cheese. Toss the ingredients together with the dressing and serve.

Per serving: Cal 301; Net Carbs 7.5g; Fat 24g; Protein 9g

Bacon & Gorgonzola Salad

Ingredients for 4 servings

- 1 ½ cups gorgonzola cheese, crumbled
- 1 head lettuce, separated into leaves
- 4 oz bacon
- 1 tbsp white wine vinegar
- 3 tbsp extra virgin olive oil
- Salt and black pepper to taste
- 2 tbsp pumpkin seeds

Directions and Total Time: approx. 15 minutes

Cut the bacon into bite-sized pieces. Fry in a skillet on medium heat for 6 minutes until golden and crispy. Mix the olive oil, white wine vinegar, salt, and pepper in a small bowl until you have a well-combined dressing. Assemble the salad by placing the lettuce on a platter and topping it with the bacon or gorgonzola cheese. To serve, drizzle the dressing on the salad and toss it.

Per serving: Cal 339; Net Carbs 3g; Fat 32g; Protein 16g

Spiced Pumpkin Soup

Prep time: 15 mins., cook time: 50 min., total time: 65 min.

Serves: 4

Ingredients:

- 3 tbsp. butter
- $\frac{1}{4}$ medium onion, chopped
- 2 cloves garlic, roasted, minced
- $\frac{1}{2}$ tsp fresh ginger
- 1 cup pumpkin puree
- 2 cups chicken broth
- 4 slices bacon
- $\frac{1}{2}$ cup heavy cream

Spices:

- 1 tsp crumbled bay leaf
- $\frac{1}{8}$ tsp nutmeg
- $\frac{1}{4}$ tsp coriander
- $\frac{1}{4}$ tsp cinnamon
- $\frac{1}{2}$ tsp freshly minced ginger
- $\frac{1}{2}$ tsp freshly ground pepper
- $\frac{1}{4}$ tsp salt

Instructions:

Heat the butter in large saucepan over medium heat. Once the butter has melted, add the ginger, garlic and onion. Saute until onions become translucent (about three minutes). Mix all the spices together in a small bowl. Set aside the pumpkin puree. Stir the spices for 2 minutes in the translucent oil. Mix in the chicken broth. Bring mixture to a boil on low heat for 20 minutes. Blend all ingredients until smooth. Continue cooking for 20 minutes. While waiting, use medium heat to cook the bacon. Once the soup is smooth, add the heavy cream and the liquid left over from the bacon. Add the bacon crumbles to the soup.

Nutritional information:

Calories 371, fat 30.7g, cholesterol 86mg, sodium 1382mg, carbs. 10.5g, dietary fiber 2.9g, sugars 3.6g, protein 14.4g

Green Squash Salad

Ingredients for 4 servings

- 2 tbsp butter
- 2 lb green squash, cubed
- 1 fennel bulb, sliced
- 2 oz chopped green onions
- 1 cup mayonnaise
- 2 tbsp chives, finely chopped
- 2 tbsp chopped dill
- A pinch of mustard powder

Directions and Total Time: approx. 15 minutes

Heat butter in a saucepan on medium heat. Let squash cook until softened (about 7 minutes). Mix squash, fennel and green onions in a bowl. Add mayonnaise, mustard powder, chives and mustard powder. Add dill to the dish.

Per serving: Cal 321; Net Carbs 9g; Fat 31g; Protein 4g

Chicken Enchilada Soup

Prep time: 10 mins., cook time: 50 min., total time: 60 min,

Serves: 4

Ingredients:

- 6 stalks celery, diced
- 1 medium red bell pepper
- 2 tsp minced garlic
- $\frac{1}{2}$ cup chopped cilantro
- $\frac{1}{4}$ tsp salt

- $\frac{1}{4}$ tsp freshly ground pepper
- 4 cups tomatoes, diced
- 7 cups chicken broth
- 6 oz. Cream cheese
- 7 oz. Shredded chicken
- 4 oz. Cream cheese
- Juice of 1 lime

Instructions:

For 3 minutes, saute celery, pepper, and garlic in hot oil on medium heat in a pot. Mix the spices for 1 minute. Add the chicken broth and the cilantro to the bowl. Boil the soup. Allow it to simmer for 20 minutes. Stir in the cream cheese. Boil the soup again and simmer for 20 more minutes. Stir the soup well and add the lime juice and shredded chicken. Serve with low-carb crackers.

Nutritional information:

Calories 344, fat 19.3g, cholesterol 85mg, sodium 1671mg, carbs. 15.1g, dietary fiber 3.6g, sugars 8.2g, protein 28.4g

Chorizo & Tomato Salad with Olives

Ingredients for 4 servings

- 2 tbsp olive oil
- 4 chorizo sausages, chopped
- 2 ½ cups cherry tomatoes
- 2 tsp red wine vinegar
- 1 small red onion, chopped
- 2 tbsp chopped cilantro
- 8 sliced Kalamata olives
- 1 head Boston lettuce, shredded
- Salt and black pepper to taste

Directions and Total Time: approx. 10 minutes

In a large skillet, heat 1 tablespoon olive oil and fry the chorizo until golden. Cut in half cherry tomatoes. Mix the olive oil, vinegar, salt and pepper in a bowl. Toss in the chopped lettuce, onions, tomatoes, cilantro, and Chorizo. Serve with olives.

Per serving: Cal 211; Net Carbs 5.2g; Fat 17g; Protein 10g

Cauliflower Soup With Roasted Red Bell Pepper

Prep time: 20 mins., cook time: 60 min., total time: 80 min.

Serves: 4

Ingredients:

- 2 medium red bell peppers, halved and de-seeded
- $\frac{1}{2}$ head cauliflower, split in florets
- 4 tbsp. Duck fat, melted
- $\frac{1}{4}$ tsp salt
- $\frac{1}{4}$ tsp freshly ground pepper
- 3 medium diced green onions
- 1 tsp smoked paprika
- 1 tsp dried thyme
- 1 tsp garlic powder
- $\frac{1}{4}$ tsp red pepper flakes
- 4 scoop whey protein
- 3 oz. Crumbled goat cheese

Instructions:

Cover baking tray with foil; put the oven on broil setting and lay sliced peppers skin sideways on the baking tray; broil till pepper skin is charred and black (about 15 minutes). Cut the cauliflower into florets before the peppers broil. Cover the broiled pepper with a lid and transfer it to a container. Season cauliflower with salt and pepper. Add 2 tablespoons of olive oil. Melted duck fat; roast at 450 degrees for 25 minutes. Remove the skins from the peppers. The remaining duck fat can be heated and then stirred in with the green onions. Toast the seasonings in each green onion. Mix in the red pepper, fat broth, whey protein, and cauliflower. Let simmer for 20 minutes. Pulse together the mixture. Add cream and additional seasonings. Serve with goat cheese and crispy bacon.

Nutritional information:

Calories 365, fat 22.5g, cholesterol 100mg, sodium 290mg, carbs. 12.4g, dietary fiber 2.3g, sugars 5.7g, protein 30.3g

Tomato & Colby Cheese Salad

Ingredients for 2 servings

- ½ cucumber, sliced
- 2 tomatoes, sliced
- ½ yellow bell pepper, sliced
- ½ red onion, sliced thinly
- ½ cup Colby cheese, cubed
- 10 green olives, pitted
- ½ tbsp red wine vinegar
- 4 tbsp olive oil
- ½ tsp dried oregano Salt and black pepper to serve

Directions and Total Time: approx. 10 minutes

In a bowl, combine the tomatoes, bell peppers, cucumbers, Colby cheese, and red onion. Toss the ingredients in a bowl with olive oil and red wine vinegar. Season with salt and pepper. Serve with olives.

Per serving: Cal 398; Net Carbs 2.4g; Fat 41g; Protein 9g

Sausage-Pepper Soup

Prep time: 15 mins., cook time: 55 min., total time: 70 min.

Serves: 4

Ingredients:

- 1 tbsp. Olive oil
- 3 lbs. Pork sausage, thickly sliced
- 1 medium green bell pepper
- 1 tsp chili powder
- 1 tsp cumin
- 1 tsp garlic powder
- $\frac{1}{4}$ tsp. Salt
- $\frac{1}{4}$ tsp freshly ground pepper
- 1 cup chopped tomatoes
- 5 oz. Raw spinach
- $\frac{1}{2}$ tsp Italian seasoning

Instructions:

Saute the sausage in olive oil over medium heat. Sear the sausage on both sides. Cook the sausage for 7 minutes. Once the spinach is soft, stir in the broth and sausage. Cover and cook covered for 30 minutes on medium-low heat. Cover and continue to simmer for 15 minutes.

Nutritional information:

Calories 812, fat 67.1g, cholesterol 191mg, sodium 1821mg, carbs. 4.4g, dietary fiber 1.4g, sugars 2.1g, protein 45.4g

Cranberry & Tempeh Broccoli Salad

Ingredients for 4 servings
- 1 lb broccoli florets
- ¾ lb tempeh, cubed
- 2 tbsp butter
- 2 tbsp almonds
- ½ cup frozen cranberries
- Salt and black pepper to taste

Directions and Total Time: approx. 15 minutes

Heat butter in a large skillet. Once the butter has melted, heat oil and fry the tempeh cubes on both sides. Stir-fry the broccoli for 6 minutes. Season with salt & pepper. Turn off the heat. To warm the salad, stir in the almonds and cranberries. Divide the salad among bowls, and then serve.

Per serving: Cal 278; Net Carbs 9g; Fat 18g; Protein 12g

The Drop Soup

Prep time: 5 mins., cook time: 5 min., total time: 10 min.

Serves: 4

Ingredients:
- 2 cups chicken broth
- 1 tbsp. Chicken bouillon, 1/2 cubed
- 1 tbsp. Butter
- 1 tbsp. Garlic paste
- 2 eggs, large

Instructions:

Place the butter in a saucepan and heat on medium heat. Add the butter, chicken broth, and bouillon cube. Boil the mixture, then stir in the garlic paste. Turn off the heat. In the boiling broth, stir the eggs and simmer for 5 minutes.

Nutritional information:

Calories 306, fat 23.1g, cholesterol 358mg, sodium 1866mg, carbs. 3.6g, dietary fiber 0g, sugars 2.2g, protein 21g

Lettuce, Beet & Tofu Salad

Ingredients for 4 servings
- 2 tbsp butter
- 2 oz tofu, cubed
- 8 oz red beets, washed
- ½ red onion, sliced
- 1 cup mayonnaise
- 1 small romaine lettuce, torn
- 2 tbsp freshly chopped chives
- Salt and black pepper to taste

Directions and Total Time: approx. 55 minutes

Place the beets on a saucepan over medium heat. Cover with salted water and bring to boil for 40 minutes, or until they are soft. Let cool. Drain. Take off the skin and cut the beets. Heat butter in a saucepan over medium heat. Fry tofu for 3-4 minutes. Transfer to a plate. Mix beets with tofu, red onions, lettuce, salt and pepper in a bowl. Serve with chives.

Per serving: Cal 315; Net Carbs 6g; Fat 30g; Protein 7g

Mixed Green Salad

Prep time: 5 mins., cook time: 7 min., total time: 7 min,

Serves: 4

Ingredients:
- 2 medium slices bacon, cooked
- 2 oz. Mixed greens
- 2 tbsp. Shaved parmesan
- 3 tbsp. Roasted pine nuts

- $\frac{1}{4}$ tsp salt
- $\frac{1}{4}$ tsp freshly ground pepper

Instructions:

Boil bacon until crispy. Layer the greens in an open container that you can shake well without spilling any of the contents. Mix the bacon pieces and all the ingredients together in a container. Shake vigorously to coat everything evenly.

Nutritional information:

Calories 142, fat 9.5g, cholesterol 26mg, sodium 775mg, carbs. 4.2g, dietary fiber 1.3g, sugars 0.9g, protein 9.9g

Cream Soup with Avocado & Zucchini

Ingredients for 4 servings
- 3 tsp vegetable oil
- 1 leek, chopped
- ½ rutabaga, sliced
- 3 cups zucchinis, chopped
- 1 avocado, chopped
- Salt and black pepper to taste
- 4 cups vegetable broth
- 2 tbsp fresh mint, chopped

Directions and Total Time: approx. 40 minutes

Warm the vegetable oil in a pot over medium heat. Saute the leek, and zucchini for 7-10 minutes. Season the dish with salt and pepper. Bring to boil broth. Reduce heat to medium and simmer for 20 mins. Remove from heat. Add the soup and avocado in batches to a blender. Blend until smooth and creamy. Add mint to the mixture and mix well.

Per serving: Cal 278; Net Carbs 9.3g; Fat 20g; Protein 8g

Sausage And Pepper Soup

SERVES 6
INGREDIENTS

- 30 oz. pork sausage
- 1 tbsp. olive oil
- 10 oz. raw spinach
- 1 medium green bell pepper
- 1 can tomatoes with jalapeños
- 4 cups beef stock
- 1 tbsp. onion powder
- 1 tbsp. chili powder
- 1 tsp. cumin garlic powder
- 1 tsp. Italian seasoning
- Salt

Directions

Heat the olive oil on a medium heat. Once the oil is hot, add the sausage and stir. Stir. Add the chopped green pepper to the pot. Stir well. Season with salt & pepper. Mix in the tomatoes and jalapenos. Stir. Cover the pot with the spinach. Once the spinach is wilted add the broth and spices. Cook the soup for 30 minutes more. Cover the pot and heat on medium-low. When it is done, remove the lid and let the soup simmer for around 10 minutes.

Nutritional Info Per Serving

Calories: 525 Fat: 45g Net Carbs: 4g Protein: 28g

Chinese Tofu Soup

Ingredients for 2 servings
- 2 cups chicken stock
- 1 tbsp soy sauce, sugar-free
- 2 spring onions, sliced
- 1 tsp sesame oil, softened
- 2 eggs, beaten
- 1-inch piece ginger, grated
- Salt and black pepper to taste
- ½ lb extra-firm tofu, cubed
- 1 tbsp fresh cilantro, chopped

Directions and Total Time: approx. 15 minutes

Boil the mixture in a saucepan over medium heat. Add soy sauce, chicken broth, and sesame oil. As you mix, add eggs. Turn heat down to low, and then add spring onions, black pepper, and ginger. Cook for 5 minutes. Tofu should be placed in a saucepan and allowed to simmer for about 1 to 2 minutes. Divide among soup bowls and garnish with fresh cilantro.

Per serving: Cal 213; Net Carbs 4.4g; Fat 15g;

Protein 18g

Caprese Salad

SERVES 2

Ingredients

- 1 tomato
- 6 oz. fresh mozzarella cheese
- ¼ cup chopped fresh basil
- 3 tbsp. olive oil
- Freshly cracked black pepper
- Salt

Directions

Place the fresh basil in a food processor with some oil. Blend the mixture until it becomes a paste. Chop the mozzarella and slice the tomatoes. Place the mozzarella and basil paste on top of each tomato. Season the dish with olive oil, black pepper, and salt.

Nutritional Info Per Serving

Calories: 407 Fat: 38g Net Carbs: 3.7g Protein: 16g

Summer Gazpacho with Cottage Cheese

Ingredients for 4 servings

- 1 green pepper, roasted
- 1 red pepper, roasted
- 1 avocado, flesh scoped out
- 1 garlic clove
- 1 spring onion, chopped
- 1 cucumber, chopped
- ½ cup olive oil
- 1 tbsp lemon juice
- 2 tomatoes, chopped
- 4 oz cottage cheese, crumbled
- 1 small red onion, chopped
- 1 tbsp apple cider vinegar
- Salt to taste

Directions and Total Time: approx. 15 min + cooling time

Blend the bell peppers, tomatoes and red onions with the lemon juice, olive oil, vinegar and half of the cucumber. Add 1 cup water. Blend until you achieve the desired consistency. Adjust the seasoning. Transfer the mixture into a large pot. Cover the mixture and let it chill in the refrigerator for at least two hours. Top the soup with the rest of the cucumber, spring onions, and a drizzle of extra olive oil.

Per serving: Cal 373; Net Carbs 8g; Fat 34g; Protein 6g

Asian Salad

SERVES 1

INGREDIENTS

- 1 packet shirataki noodles
- 2 tbsp. coconut oil
- 1 cucumber
- 1 spring onion
- ¼ tbsp. red pepper flakes
- 1 tbsp. sesame oil
- 1 tbsp. rice vinegar
- 1 tsp. sesame seeds
- Salt and pepper

DIRECTIONS

Rinse the shirataki noodles. Take out all excess water. Let the noodles dry on a towel. Heat the coconut oil in a saucepan on medium heat. Fry the noodles for about 5-7 minutes. Set aside to cool on a towel. Peel and slice the cucumber. Place the cucumber on a plate and then add the rest of your ingredients. Sprinkle the cucumber with the remaining ingredients. Allow to chill in the refrigerator for 30 minutes. Serve with fried shirataki pasta.

NUTRITIONAL INFO PER SERVING

Calories: 418

Fat: 45g

Net Carbs: 8g

Protein: 3g

Fresh Avocado-Cucumber Soup

Ingredients for 4 servings

- 3 tbsp olive oil
- 1 small onion, chopped
- 4 large cucumbers, chopped

- 1 avocado, peeled and pitted
- Salt and black pepper to taste
- 1 ½ cups water
- ½ cup Greek yogurt
- 1 tbsp cilantro, chopped
- 2 limes, juiced
- 1 garlic clove, minced
- 1 tomato, chopped

Directions and Total Time: approx. 10 min + cooling time

Place all ingredients except the avocado and tomato into a food processor. Blend for 2 minutes, or until smooth. Place the mixture in a bowl. Cover the bowl and let it rest for at least 2 hours in the refrigerator. Add avocado and tomatoes.

Per serving: Cal 243; Net Carbs 9.3g; Fat 20g; Protein 5g

Summer Tomato Soup

(Ready in about 40 min | Servings 4)

Per serving: 202 Calories; 16.1g Fat; 7g Carbs; 1.8g Fiber; 6g Protein

Ingredients

- 2 cloves garlic, finely sliced
- 1/2 large red onion, finely chopped
- 2 tablespoons olive oil
- salt and pepper, to taste
- 1 ½ tablespoon tomato paste
- 2 cups tomatoes, peeled and diced
- 2 celery stalks, peeled and chopped
- 2 cups vegetable broth
- 1/3 teaspoon paprika
- 1/3 teaspoon oregano
- ½ cup heavy cream
- ½ teaspoon dried basil
- ½ cup parmesan cheese, shredded

Directions

In a large saucepan, heat the olive oil. Add the celery, garlic, and red onions. Cook for about 2 minutes. Stir in the tomato paste, vegetable broth, and tomatoes. Season with salt, pepper, paprika, oregano, and basil. Boil the tomatoes for between 20 and 25 minutes, or until they are soft. Blend the mixture with an immersion blender. Continue to boil the heavy cream for about 1-2 minutes. Serve in bowls, and garnish with parmesan cheese.

Zuppa Toscana with Kale

Ingredients for 4 servings

- 2 cups chicken broth
- 1 tbsp olive oil
- ¼ cup heavy cream
- 1 cup kale
- 3 oz pancetta, chopped
- 1 parsnip, chopped
- 1 garlic clove, minced
- Salt and black pepper to taste
- ¼ tsp red pepper flakes
- ½ onion, chopped
- 1 lb hot Italian sausage, sliced
- 2 tbsp Parmesan, grated

Directions and Total Time: approx. 40 minutes

Heat the olive oil in a pan on medium heat. Stir-fry the sausage, garlic, onion, and pancetta for five minutes. Stir in the chicken broth and parsnip, and let simmer for about 15-20 minutes. Mix in all remaining ingredients except the Parmesan cheese and simmer for 5 minutes. Sprinkle with Parmesan cheese.

Per serving: Cal 543; Net Carbs 5.6g; Fat 45g; Protein 45g

Easy Green Baby Spinach Soup

(Ready in about 25 min | Servings 6)

Per serving: 173 Calories; 18g Fat; 3g Carbs; 1g Protein

Ingredients

- 5 cups spinach
- 2 small onions, finely chopped
- 2 medium-size carrots, finely chopped
- ½ cups coconut oil
- 2 garlic cloves, sliced
- 1 teaspoon pepper
- 1 teaspoon salt
- 12 cups water
- 1 cube vegetable broth
- ½ cup parmesan cheese, grated

Directions

In a large saucepan, heat the coconut oil. Add the onion, carrot, and garlic. Let it simmer for three minutes. Next, add the water and vegetable broth. Bring to boil for 8 minutes. Add the spinach to the saucepan and continue boiling for 12 minutes. Season the soup with salt and pepper. Blend the soup in a blender until smooth. Use small batches. Serve warm and sprinkle with parmesan cheese. Enjoy!

Awesome Chicken Enchilada Soup

Ingredients for 4 servings

- ½ lb boneless, skinless chicken thighs
- 2 tbsp coconut oil
- ¾ cup red enchilada sauce
- 1 onion, chopped
- 3 oz canned diced green chilis
- 1 avocado, sliced
- 1 cup cheddar, shredded
- 1 pickled jalapeño, chopped
- ½ cup sour cream
- 1 tomato, diced

Directions and Total Time: approx. 35 minutes

Put a large pan over medium heat. Heat coconut oil. Cook the chicken until golden brown on the outside. Cook for 2 minutes. Stir in the onion, jalapeno and green chilis. Add 4 cups water and enchilada sauce. Let the chicken simmer for 20 minutes. Place the soup in a bowl. Top it with the cheese, sour milk, tomato, avocado, and a drizzle of olive oil.

Per serving: Cal 543; Net Carbs 8.7g; Fat 44g; Protein 28g

Greek Cucumber Salad with Yogurt

(Ready in about 15 min | Servings 4)

Per serving: 122 Calories; 6.2g Fat; 6g Carbs; 1.8g Fiber; 9.5g Protein

Ingredients

- 1 ½ cup plain Greek yogurt
- 3 cucumbers, peeled and cut into small cubes
- 1 ½ tablespoon olive oil
- ½ teaspoon salt

- 2 tablespoons fresh dill, chopped
- 2 garlic cloves, minced
- 1/3 teaspoon ground pepper
- ¼ cup mint leaves, for garnish

Directions

Combine the Greek yogurt, minced garlic and cucumber in a large bowl. Add the fresh dill. Combine all ingredients. Mix well. Drizzle olive oil over the mixture and season with salt, pepper, and freshly ground black pepper. Allow to cool for 30 minutes, then serve with fresh mint leaves.

Cauliflower Soup with Crispy Bacon

Ingredients for 4 servings
- 2 tbsp olive oil
- 1 onion, chopped
- ¼ celery root, grated
- 10 oz cauliflower florets
- Salt and black pepper to taste
- 1 cup almond milk
- 1 cup white cheddar, shredded
- 2 oz bacon, cut into strips

Directions and Total Time: approx. 25 minutes

Fry the bacon in a skillet on medium heat for 5 minutes. Transfer to a plate lined with paper towels. Warm olive oil in the same skillet and saute onion for 3 minutes to make it fragrant. Saute the celery root, cauliflower florets, and celery root for 3 minutes. Season the mixture with salt and pepper. Bring to boil and reduce heat to low. Cover and cook for 10 minutes. Blend the soup using an immersion blender until all ingredients are well combined. Add the almond milk, cheese, and stir until the cheese melts. Salt and pepper to taste. Serve hot with crispy bacon.

Per serving: Cal 323; Net Carbs 7.6g; Fat 27g; Protein 13g

Cauliflower Soup with Bacon

(Ready in about 40 minutes | Servings 6)

Per serving: 151 Calories; 13g Fat; 5.4g Carbs; 1.5g Fiber; 2.4g Protein

Ingredients

- 1 medium head cauliflower, cut into florets
- 2 tablespoons olive oil
- 3 cups vegetable broth
- 1 onion, chopped
- 2 cloves garlic, minced
- 1/3 cup heavy cream
- salt and pepper, to taste
- 1 teaspoon dried oregano
- 1 teaspoon thyme
- 2 tablespoons butter
- 1/3 cup cooked bacon

Directions

Preheat your oven to 400 F.

Spread the onion, garlic, and cauliflower on a baking sheet covered with baking paper. Use olive oil to drizzle the mixture. Season with salt & pepper. Bake the cauliflower for 20 minutes or until it is tender. In a soup pot, combine the cauliflower, onion, and garlic. Add the butter, vegetable broth and thyme to the pot. Season with salt, pepper, and thyme. Mix well, and boil for 15 minutes. Let the soup cool down for a while before transferring it to a blender. Blend in the cream until smooth. Use small batches. Garnish with bacon.

Reuben Soup

Ingredients for 4 servings

- 1 parsnip, chopped
- 1 onion, diced
- 3 cups beef stock
- 1 celery stalk, diced
- 1 garlic clove, minced
- 1 cup heavy cream
- ½ cup sauerkraut, shredded
- ½ lb corned beef, chopped
- 2 tbsp lard
- ½ cup mozzarella, shredded
- Salt and black pepper to taste Chopped chives for garnish

Directions and Total Time: approx. 30 minutes

In a large saucepan, melt the lard. Stir in the parsnip, onion and garlic. Fry for 3 minutes, until tender. Stir in the beef stock and sauerkraut. Bring to boil. Turn down the heat and add the corned meat. Allow to cook for 15 minutes. Adjust the seasoning. Mix in heavy cream and cheese, and let it cook for about 1 minute. Serve with chopped

chives.

Per serving: Cal 363; Net Carbs 5g; Fat 21g; Protein 21g

Mushroom Cream Soup with Herbs

Ingredients for 4 servings

- 12 oz white mushrooms, chopped
- 1 onion, chopped
- ½ cup heavy cream
- ¼ cup butter
- 1 tsp thyme leaves, chopped
- 1 tsp parsley leaves, chopped
- 1 tsp cilantro leaves, chopped
- 2 garlic cloves, minced
- 4 cups vegetable broth
- Salt and black pepper to taste

Directions and Total Time: approx. 25 minutes

Heat the butter in large saucepan over high heat. Add the garlic and onion to the pot and cook for 3 minutes. Stir-fry the mushrooms with salt and pepper for 5 minutes. Bring to a boil the broth. Reduce heat to low and simmer for 10 minutes. Blend soup using a hand blender until smooth. Add heavy cream. Add herbs.

Per serving: Cal 232; Net Carbs 6.4g; Fat 20g; Protein 8g

Garden Zucchini Soup

(Ready in about 15 min | Servings 5)

Per serving: 154 Calories; 10.1g Fat; 6.8g Carbs; 0.8g Fiber; 6.9g Protein

Ingredients

- 4 medium zucchini, diced
- 1 large yellow onion, chopped
- 2 cloves garlic, sliced
- salt and pepper, to taste
- 2 tablespoons butter
- 4 cups vegetable broth
- 1 cup parmesan cheese, grated
- ½ teaspoon dried rosemary
- ½ teaspoon dried basil

Directions

Melt the butter in a large pot, saute the garlic and

onion for 3 minutes. Add the zucchini diced and cook for 8-9 mins. Add the vegetable broth, and cook for about 12 minutes, or until zucchini is soft. Remove the pot from the stove and add salt, pepper, dried basil and rosemary. Puree with an immersion blender until smooth. Serve hot and sprinkle with parmesan cheese.

Curried Shrimp & Green Bean Soup

Ingredients for 4 servings

- 1 onion, chopped
- 2 tbsp red curry paste
- 2 tbsp butter
- 1 lb jumbo shrimp, deveined
- 2 tsp ginger-garlic puree
- 1 cup coconut milk Salt and chili pepper to taste
- 1 bunch green beans, halved
- 1 tbsp cilantro, chopped

Directions and Total Time: approx. 20 minutes

Add the shrimp to the melted butter in a pan over medium-high heat. Season with salt and pepper and cook until opaque for about 2 to 3 minutes. Transfer them to the plate. Mix the ginger-garlic puree onion and red curry paste. Saute for two minutes until fragrant. Mix in the coconut milk, and then add shrimp, salt, chili pepper and green beans. Cook for four minutes. Reduce the temperature to a simmer, and cook for an additional 3 minutes, while stirring. Taste the soup by adding salt. Pour the soup into serving bowls, then sprinkle with chopped cilantro.

Per serving: Cal 315; Net Carbs 4.2g; Fat 22g; Protein 25g

Hearty Fall Stew

Preparation Time: 15 minutes

Cooking Time: 8 hrs.

Servings: 6

Ingredients:

- tablespoons extra-virgin olive oil, divided
- 1 (2-pound/907-g) beef chuck roast, cut into 1-inch chunks

- 1/2 teaspoon salt
- 1/4 teaspoon freshly ground black pepper
- 1/4 cup apple cider vinegar
- 1/2 sweet onion, chopped
- 1 cup diced tomatoes
- teaspoon dried thyme
- 11/2 cups pumpkin, cut into 1-inch chunks
- 2 cups beef broth
- teaspoons minced garlic
- 1 tablespoon chopped fresh parsley, for garnish

Directions:

Add the beef to the skillet and add salt, pepper for seasoning. Roast the meat for seven minutes or until it is well-browned. Put the beef in the slow cooker. Add all the remaining ingredients, with the exception for the parsley, into in the slow cooker. Mix well. Slow cook for 8 hours. Then sprinkle with chopped parsley before serving.

Nutrition:

Calories: 462 Fat: 19.1g Fiber: 11.6g Carbohydrates: 10.7 g Protein: 18.6 g

Hearty Vegetable Soup

Ingredients for 4 servings

- 2 tsp olive oil
- 1 onion, chopped
- 1 garlic clove, minced
- ½ celery stalk, chopped
- 1 cup mushrooms, sliced
- ½ head broccoli, chopped
- ½ carrot, sliced
- 1 cup spinach, torn into pieces
- Salt and black pepper to taste
- 2 thyme sprigs, chopped
- ½ tsp dried rosemary
- 3 cups vegetable stock
- 1 tomato, chopped
- ½ cup almond milk

Directions and Total Time: approx. 35 minutes

Heat olive oil in a saucepan. Add celery, onion, carrot and garlic and cook until they are translucent with a little stirring now and then, approximately 5 minutes. Add the broccoli, mushrooms, tomatoes, salt, rosemary, pepper, thyme along with vegetable stock. Let the ingredients simmer for 15 minutes, while the lid remains open. Mix in the almond milk and spinach and cook for another 5 minutes. Serve.

Per serving: Cal 94; Net Carbs 4.9g; Fat 3g; Protein 2g

Chicken Mushroom Soup

Preparation Time: 15 minutes

Cooking Time: 10-15 minutes

Servings: 4

Ingredients:

- 6 cups of chicken stock
- 5 slices of chopped bacon
- 4 cups cooked chicken breast, chopped
- 3 cups of water
- 2 cups of chopped celery root
- 2 cups of sliced yellow squash
- 2 tablespoons of olive oil
- 1/2 teaspoon of avocado oil
- 1/4 cup of chopped basil
- 1/4 cup of chopped onion
- 1/4 cup of chopped tomatoes
- 1 tablespoon of ground garlic
- 1 cup of sliced white mushrooms
- 1 cup green beans
- Salt
- Black pepper

Directions:

In a skillet, heat the oil and add one-half of onions and saute until soft. In the bacon, cook for about one-half minutes. After that, add onions, garlic, tomatoes and mushrooms. Stir and cook for 3 minutes. Add the fat water and stock together with the remaining ingredients. It should simmer for about 10 minutes. Serve hot.

Nutrition:

Calories: 268 Fat: 10.5g Fiber: 4.9g Carbohydrates: 3.1 g Protein: 12.9g

Tomato Cream Soup with Basil

Ingredients for 4 servings

- 1 carrot, chopped
- 2 tbsp olive oil
- 1 onion, diced
- 1 garlic clove, minced
- ¼ cup raw cashew nuts, diced
- 14 oz canned tomatoes
- 1 tsp fresh basil leaves
- Salt and black pepper to taste
- 1 cup crème fraîche

Directions and Total Time: approx. 25 minutes

In a saucepan, warm olive oil saucepan at medium-low heat. Saute the carrot, onion, and garlic for four minutes, until softened. Add the tomatoes and 2 cups water, and add the black pepper and salt. Cover and simmer for 10 minutes or until the tomatoes are completely cooked. Blend the ingredients using the aid of an immersion blender. Adjust according to your taste and mix in the cashew and creme fraiche nuts. Serve with basil.

Per serving: Cal 311; Net Carbs 8g; Fat 30g; Protein 4g

Cold Green Beans and Avocado Soup

Preparation Time: 15 minutes

Cooking Time: 15 minutes

Servings: 4

Ingredients:

- tbsp. butter
- tbsp. almond oil
- 1 garlic clove, minced
- 1 cup (227 g) green beans (fresh or frozen)
- 1/4 avocado
- 1 cup heavy cream
- 1/2 cup grated cheddar cheese + extra for garnish
- 1/2 tsp. coconut aminos
- Salt to taste

Directions:

Warm the almond oil and butter in a large pan and saute in the garlic 30 secs. In the meantime, add green beans, and stir-fry for 10 minutes or until they are tender. Transfer the mix to the food processor. Top with avocados, the heavy cream, coconut aminos, cheddar cheese and salt. Blend the ingredients until smooth. Serve the soup in bowls for serving cover with plastic wraps, and then place in the refrigerator to chill for at least two hours. After that, enjoy it with a sprinkle of white cheddar cheese.

Nutrition:

Calories: 301 Fat: 3.1g Fiber: 11.5g Carbohydrates: 2.8 g Protein: 3.1g

Sausage & Turnip Soup

Ingredients for 4 servings
- 3 turnips, chopped
- 2 celery sticks, chopped
- 2 tbsp butter
- 1 tbsp olive oil
- 1 pork sausage, sliced
- 2 cups vegetable broth
- ½ cup sour cream
- 3 green onions, chopped
- Salt and black pepper to taste

Directions and Total Time: approx. 40 minutes

Saute green onions in melted butter over medium heat until soft and golden, about 3 minutes. Add turnip and celery, and cook for 5 minutes. Pour the vegetable broth and 2 cups of water over. Bring it to a boil, then cook for 20 minutes or until the vegetables are soft. Remove the soup from the cooking. Blend the soup using the aid of a hand blender until it is smooth. Add the sour cream and alter the seasoning. Heat your olive oil over a pan. Add the pork sausage and cook for five minutes. Serve the soup with pork sausage.

Per serving: Cal 215; Net Carbs 6g; Fat 20g; Protein 7g

Creamy Mixed Seafood Soup

Preparation Time: 15 minutes

Cooking Time: 15 minutes

Servings: 4

Ingredients:
- tbsp. avocado oil
- garlic cloves, minced
- 3/4 tbsp. almond flour
- 1 cup vegetable broth
- 1 tsp. dried dill
- lb. frozen mixed seafood
- Salt and black pepper to taste
- 1 tbsp. plain vinegar
- cups cooking cream
- Fresh dill leaves to garnish

Directions:

Heat oil and sauté the garlic for 30 second intervals or until it becomes fragrant. Mix in the almond flour and cook until it turns brown. Mix in the vegetable broth until smooth and stir in the dill, seafood mix, salt, and black pepper. Bring the soup to a boil and then simmer for 3 to 4 minutes or until the seafood cooks. Add the vinegar, the cooking cream and stir. Serve with dill.

Nutrition:

Calories: 361 Fat: 12.4g Fiber: 8.5g Carbohydrates:3.9 g Protein: 11.7g

Cauliflower Cheese Soup

Ingredients for 4 servings
- ½ head cauliflower, chopped
- 2 tbsp coconut oil
- ½ cup leeks, chopped
- 1 celery stalk, chopped
- 1 serrano pepper, chopped
- 1 tsp garlic puree
- 1 ½ tbsp flaxseed meal
- 1 ½ cups coconut milk
- 6 oz Monterey Jack, shredded
- Salt and black pepper to taste
- Fresh parsley, chopped

Directions and Total Time: approx. 25 minutes

In a large skillet over medium-high heat, melt the coconut oil. Then, saute the serrano pepper, celery and leeks until they are soft in approximately 5 minutes. Add coconut milk, cauliflower, 2 cups water and flaxseed meal. While covered partially, allow simmering for 10 minutes or until cooked through. Blend using your immersion blender to make it is smooth. Add the cheese shredded and mix until the cheese is fully melting and you've got a homogenous mix. Sprinkle with salt and pepper according to your preference. Decorate with chopped parsley, Serve warm.

Per serving: Cal 472; Net Carbs 7g; Fat 43g; Protein 13g

Roasted Tomato and Cheddar Soup

Preparation Time: 10 minutes

Cooking Time: 15-20 minutes

Servings: 4

Ingredients:

- 2 tbsp. butter
- 2 medium yellow onions, sliced
- 4 garlic cloves, minced
- 5 thyme sprigs
- 8 basil leaves + extra for garnish
- 8 tomatoes
- 1/2 tsp. red chili flakes
- 2 cups vegetable broth
- Salt and black pepper to taste
- 1 cup grated cheddar cheese (white and sharp)

Directions:

Melt the butter in a pot and saute the onions and garlic for 3 minutes or until softened. Add the thyme, tomatoes, basil and red chili flakes along with vegetable broth. Add the black pepper and salt. Boil the water, then let it allow to simmer 10 minutes, or till the tomatoes become soft. Puree all ingredients until smooth. Season. Sprinkle with Basil and cheddar cheese. Serve warm.

Nutrition:

Calories: 341 Fat: 12.9g Fiber: 9.6g Carbohydrates: 4.8 g Protein: 4.1g

Cheese Cream Soup with Chicken

Ingredients for 4 servings

- 2 cups cooked and shredded chicken
- 1 carrot, chopped
- 1 onion, chopped
- 3 tbsp butter
- 4 cups chicken broth
- 2 tbsp cilantro, chopped
- 1/3 cup buffalo sauce
- ½ cup cream cheese
- Salt and black pepper to taste

Directions and Total Time: approx. 20 minutes

In a skillet on medium-high heat, melt butter and cook carrots and onion until soft in approximately 5 minutes. Add the chicken and broth and heat until hot but do not bring to a boil. Sprinkle with salt and pepper. Add cream cheese and buffalo sauce and cook until it is heated through approximately 2 to 3 minutes. Serve with garnishes of cilantro.

Per serving: Cal 487; Net Carbs 5.2g; Fat 41g; Protein 16g

Cauliflower Kale Soup

Preparation Time: 10 minutes

Cooking Time: 50 minutes

Servings: 4

Ingredients:

- 4 cups cauliflower florets
- 6 cups vegetable stock
- 1 tbsp. garlic, minced
- 1/4 cup onion, chopped
- 6 oz kale, chopped
- 6 tbsp. olive oil
- Pepper Salt

Directions:

Preheat the oven until 425° F. Spread cauliflower onto the baking sheet and drizzle it with 2 tablespoons of oil. Season with salt and pepper. Roast the cauliflower in the preheated oven for about 25 minutes. Remove the cauliflower from the oven and place aside. Within a bowl mix the kale in two tablespoons of oil. Then, season with salt. Place kale on the baking sheet and cook to 300 F for 30 minutes. Toss halfway through. Cook oil. Add onion and sauté in 3-4 minutes. Add garlic and sauté for one minute. Add the cauliflower and stock and bring it to a boil. Cook in a simmer for about 10 minutes. Add kale, and cook for another 10 minutes. Blend the soup until it is smooth. Serve and enjoy.

Nutrition:

Calories: 287 Fat: 15.1g Fiber: 4.1g Carbohydrates: 3.1 g Protein: 5.8g

Cheesy Chicken Soup with Spinach

Ingredients for 4 servings
- 2 tbsp olive oil
- 1 onion, chopped
- 2 garlic cloves, minced
- 1 carrot, chopped
- 1 celery stalk, chopped
- 1 chicken breast, cubed
- 1 cup spinach
- 4 cups chicken broth
- 1 cup cheddar, shredded
- ½ tsp chili powder
- ½ tsp ground cumin
- Salt and black pepper to taste

Directions and Total Time: approx. 45 minutes

Heat the olive oil inside a pan at medium-high heat, and cook the chicken for about 3 minutes. Stir-fry in the garlic, onion and celery and carrots in 5 mins until vegetables become soft. Sprinkle with chili powder along with cumin, salt and pepper. Add the chicken broth and bring to a boil. Simmer for 15-20 minutes. Mix in the spinach to cook 5-6 mins until the spinach is wilted. Serve with cheddar cheese.

Per serving: Cal 381; Net Carbs 5.3g; Fat 28g; Protein 22g

Healthy Celery Soup

Preparation Time: 10 minutes

Cooking Time: 20 minutes

Servings: 4

Ingredients:

- 3 cups celery, chopped
- 1 cup vegetable broth
- 5 oz cream cheese
- 1 1/2 tbsp. fresh basil, chopped
- 1/4 cup onion, chopped
- tbsp. garlic, chopped
- 1 tbsp. olive oil
- 1/4 tsp. pepper
- 1/2 tsp. salt

Directions:

Warm some oil. Add celery, onion as well as garlic, to the pan and cook for about 4-5 minutes or until soft. Add broth and bring to boil. Lower heat and let it simmer. Add the cream cheese and basil to stir till cheese has melting. Season soup with pepper and salt. Puree the soup until smooth. Serve and enjoy.

Nutrition:

Calories: 201 Fat: 5.4g Fiber: 8.1g Carbohydrates: 3.9 g Protein: 5.1g

Zucchini & Leek Turkey Soup

Ingredients for 4 servings
- 2 cups turkey meat, cooked and chopped
- 1 onion, chopped
- 1 garlic clove, minced
- 3 celery stalks, chopped
- 2 leeks, chopped
- 2 tbsp butter
- 4 cups chicken stock
- Salt and black pepper to taste
- ¼ cup fresh parsley, chopped
- 1 large zucchini, spiralized

Directions and Total Time: approx. 40 minutes

Melt the butter in a pot over medium heat. Add the celery, leeks onion, garlic, and other vegetables in the pot and let them cook 5 mins. Add the turkey meat as well as salt, black pepper and stock. Cook to a simmer for about 20 mins. Mix in the zucchini in the meantime and let it cook down for five minutes. Serve in bowls topped with parsley.

Per serving: Cal 235; Net Carbs 9.3g; Fat 10g; Protein 23g

Creamy Asparagus Soup

Preparation Time: 10 minutes

Cooking Time: 15 minutes

Servings: 4

Ingredients:

- lbs. asparagus, cut the ends and chop into 1/2-inch pieces
- 2 tbsp. olive oil
- garlic cloves, minced
- 2 oz parmesan cheese, grated
- 1/2 cup heavy cream
- 1/4 cup onion, chopped
- 4 cups vegetable stock
- Pepper
- Salt

Directions:

Heat olive oil in a large pot over medium heat. Add onions to the pot, and sauté until the onion softens. Add asparagus and sauté for a couple of minutes. Add garlic, and sauté for about a minute. Sprinkle with salt and pepper. Add stock and bring to boil. Lower heat and cook until asparagus is tender. Remove the pot from the heat and blend the soup with the immersion blender to make it becomes creamy. Bring the pot back to heat. Add cream and stir well and cook over medium heat until just soup is hot. Do not boil the soup. Add cheese and stir. Serve and have a blast.

Nutrition:

Calories: 202 Fat: 8.4g Fiber: 6.1g Carbohydrates: 3.1 g Protein: 5.3g

Tomato Soup with Parmesan Croutons

Ingredients for 6 servings

- Parmesan Croutons
- 4 tbsp butter, softened
- 4 tbsp grated Parmesan
- 3 egg whites
- 1 ¼ cups almond flour
- 2 tsp baking powder
- 5 tbsp psyllium husk powder
- Tomato Soup 3 tbsp olive oil
- 2 lb fresh ripe tomatoes
- 4 cloves garlic, peeled only
- 1 small white onion, diced
- 1 red bell pepper, diced
- 1 cup coconut cream
- ½ tsp dried rosemary
- ½ tsp dried oregano
- Salt and black pepper to taste

Directions and Total Time: approx. 1 hour 25 minutes

Preheat the oven up to 350 F. Line a baking sheet with wax paper. In a bowl, combine almond flour, baking powder, and psyllium husk powder. Add eggs with whites. Stir for 30 seconds, until well combined, but not too blended. Make 8 flat pieces from the dough. Place them on the baking sheets with enough space between each piece to allow for rising. Bake for 30 minutes. Allow the croutons to cool. Split into halves. Mix the butter and Parmesan cheese. Spread the mixture on the middle of the Croutons. Cook for five minutes. On a dish for baking include tomatoes, garlic and onion, bell pepper and drizzle olive oil. Roast the vegetables by baking them in the oven. It takes about 25 minutes, and then broil until 4 mins. Transfer the vegetables to a blender and add coconut cream, oregano, rosemary, salt and pepper. Blend until smooth. Serve with the croutons.

Per serving: Cal 329; Net Carbs 9g; Fat 31g; Protein 11g

Coconut Curry Cauliflower Soup

Preparation Time: 15 minutes

Cooking Time: 30 minutes

Servings: 4

Ingredients:

- tbsp. olive oil
- 2-3 tsp. curry powder
- 1 medium onion
- tsp. ground cumin
- 3 garlic cloves

- 1/2 tsp. turmeric powder
- 1 tsp. ginger
- 14 oz coconut milk
- 14 oz tomatoes
- 1 cup vegetable broth
- 1 cauliflower
- Salt and pepper

Directions:

Take a pot, add onions and olive oil, and place it over an oven with a medium heat to cook. After three minutes add garlic, ginger, curry powder, cumin and turmeric powder. Cook for a further 5 minutes. Add tomatoes, coconut milk, vegetables broth and cauliflower to mix well. Allow the soup to heat and then bring to boil. On a low flame cook for at least 20 mins until the cauliflower softens, blend the soup well in blenders and then heat the soup for 5 minutes. Add salt and pepper according to your preference. Serve hot soup that is seasonal and warm.

Nutrition:

Calories: 281 Fat: 8.1g Fiber: 3.8g Carbohydrates: 3.2 g Protein: 4.8g

Creamy Coconut Soup with Chicken

Ingredients for 4 servings
- 3 tbsp butter
- 1 onion, chopped
- 2 chicken breasts, chopped
- Salt and black pepper to taste
- ½ cup coconut cream
- ¼ cup celery, chopped

Directions and Total Time: approx. 25 minutes

Heat the butter in a saucepan at medium-high temperature. Saute the celery and onion for 3 minutes until they are tender. Mix in the chicken and 4 cups of water, salt and pepper. Cook in 15 mins. Mix in coconut cream. Serve warm.

Per serving: Cal 442; Net Carbs 5.1g; Fat 32g; Protein 29g

Nutmeg Pumpkin Soup

Preparation Time: 15 minutes

Cooking Time: 20 minutes

Servings: 4

Ingredients:
- 1 tablespoon of butter
- 1 onion (diced)
- 1 16-ounce can of pumpkin puree
- 1 1/3 cups of vegetable broth
- 1/2 tablespoon of nutmeg
- 1/2 tablespoon of sugar Salt (to taste)
- Pepper (to taste)
- 3 cups of soymilk or any milk as a substitute

Directions:

Using a large saucepan, add onion to margarine. Cook for 3 and 5 minutes or until the onion is translucent. Add pumpkin puree, vegetable broth, pepper, sugar, and the rest of the ingredients, and stir until well-mixed. Cook in medium heat for between 10 and fifteen minutes Before serving the soup, taste and add more spices, pepper, and salt if necessary. Serve soup and enjoy it!

Nutrition: Calories: 165 Fat: 4.9g Fiber: 11.9g Carbohydrates: 3.5 g Protein: 4.2g

Cream of Cauliflower & Leek Soup

Ingredients for 4 servings
- 4 cups vegetable broth
- 16 oz cauliflower florets
- 1 celery stalk, chopped
- 1 onion, chopped
- 1 cup leeks, chopped
- 2 tbsp butter
- 1 tbsp olive oil
- 1 cup heavy cream
- ½ tsp red pepper flakes

Directions and Total Time: approx. 45 minutes

Heat the butter, olive oil and the saucepan that is set over medium-high heat. Saute onion, leeks and celery for five minutes. Stir in the broth and cauliflower and bring to a boil; simmer for 30 minutes. Transfer the mixture to an immersion blender and puree; add in the heavy cream and stir.

Decorate with red pepper flakes and serve.

Per serving: Cal 275; Net Carbs 8.3g; Fat 21g; Protein 8g

Turkey Salad

Preparation time: **5 minutes**
Cooking time: **0 minutes**
Servings: **4**

Ingredients:

- 1 cup cherry tomatoes, halved
- 1 cucumber, sliced
- 1 carrot, grated
- Salt and black pepper to the taste
- 1 tablespoon balsamic vinegar
- 1 tablespoon olive oil
- 1 and ½ cups turkey breast, cooked, skinless, boneless and shredded

Directions:

In a salad bowl, combine the turkey, cucumber, tomatoes and other ingredients. Toss them and serve with lunch.

Nutrition: calories 57, fat 3.7, fiber 1.3, carbs 6.1, protein 1.2

Broccoli & Spinach Soup

Ingredients for 4 servings

- 2 tbsp butter
- 1 onion, chopped
- 1 garlic clove, minced
- 2 heads broccoli, cut in florets
- 2 stalks celery, chopped
- 4 cups vegetable broth
- 1 cup baby spinach
- Salt and black pepper to taste
- 1 tbsp basil, chopped Parmesan, shaved to serve

Directions and Total Time: approx. 25 minutes

Melt the butter in a saucepan over medium heat. Sauté the onion and garlic for 3 minutes, until they soften. Add the celery and broccoli, and cook for 4 minutes or until slightly tender. Add the broth and

bring it to a boil before reducing the heat to medium-low and simmer covered for approximately 5 minutes. Drop in the spinach to wilt, adjust the seasonings, and cook for 4 minutes. Ladle soup into serving bowls. Serve with a sprinkle of grated Parmesan cheese and basil.

Per serving: Cal 123; Net Carbs 3.4g; Fat 10g; Protein 6g

Cheesy Turkey Pan

Preparation time: **10 minutes**
Cooking time: **25 minutes**
Servings: **4**

Ingredients:

- 2 cups cheddar cheese, grated
- 1 big turkey breast, skinless, boneless and cubed
- 1 tablespoon tomato passata
- ¼ cup veggie stock
- 1 tablespoon olive oil
- 2 shallots, chopped
- ¼ cup tomatoes, cubed
- Salt and black pepper to the taste

Directions:

Prepare a pan by heating the oil at medium-high heat. Add the shallots, and cook for two minutes. Add the meat to the pan and cook over a medium heat for five minutes. Add the passata, as well as other ingredients, except for the cheese. Mix and cook on low heat for about 10 minutes. Sprinkle the cheese over and cook for about 7-8 minutes, then divide the dish and serve with lunch.

Nutrition: calories 309, fat 23.1, fiber 0.4, carbs 3.9, protein 21.6

Cream of Roasted Jalapeño Soup

Ingredients for 6 servings

- 3 tbsp melted butter
- 1 jalapeño pepper,
- halved 6 green bell peppers,
- halved 1 bulb garlic, halved,
- not peeled 6 tomatoes,
- halved 3 cups vegetable broth

- 2/3 cup heavy cream
- 4 tbsp grated Parmesan
- 2 tbsp chopped chives
- Salt and black pepper to taste

Directions and Total Time: approx. 45 min + cooling time

Preheat the oven at 350 F. Arrange bell peppers, jalapeno pepper as well as garlic, on a baking sheet to roast and bake for about 15 mins. Add tomatoes and cook for about 15 minutes. Cool. Peel off the skins and put them in a blender. Add salt and pepper, butter, vegetable broth and heavy cream. Blend until smooth. Transfer to a saucepan over medium-high heat, to cook 3-4 mins. Serve into bowls sprinkled with Parmesan cheese and chives.

Per serving: Cal 181; Net Carbs 9.5g; Fat 13g; Protein 5g

Chicken and Leeks Pan

Preparation time: **10 minutes**

Cooking time: **20 minutes**

Servings: **4**

Ingredients:

- 2 tablespoons olive oil
- 1 pound chicken breast, skinless, boneless and cut into strips
- 2 shallots, chopped
- 1 cup mozzarella cheese, shredded
- 2 leeks, sliced
- ½ cup veggie stock
- 1 tablespoon heavy cream
- 1 teaspoon sweet paprika
- Salt and black pepper to the taste

Directions:

In a pan, heat the oil at medium-high heat. Add the shallots stirring until they are cooked for three minutes. Add the meat, as well as the leeks. Stir and cook for another 7 minutes. Add the remaining ingredients, except for the cheese. Stir. Sprinkle the cheese over and then place the pan into the oven and cook the mixture to 400° F for 10 minutes longer. Divide the mixture between dishes and then serve.

Nutrition: calories 253, fat 12.9, fiber 1, carbs 7.2, protein 26.9

Chicken and Peppers Mix

Preparation time: **10 minutes**

Cooking time: **25 minutes**

Servings: **4**

Ingredients:

- 1 cup red bell peppers, cut into strips
- 1 pound chicken breast, skinless, boneless and roughly cubed
- 2 spring onions, chopped
- 2 tablespoons olive oil
- 1 tomato, cubed
- Salt and black pepper to the taste
- ¼ cup tomato passata
- 1 tablespoon cilantro, chopped

Directions:

Prepare a pan using the oil at medium-high heat. Add spring onions and cook for 2 minutes. Add the chicken and bell peppers. Stir and cook the mixture for an additional 8 minutes. Add the remaining ingredients, cook to an unbeatable simmer, then cook on medium heat for about 15 minutes, stirring frequently. Divide the mixture between plates and serve.

Nutrition: calories 206, fat 10, fiber 0.9, carbs 3.7, protein 24.8

Paprika Chicken Mix

Preparation time: **10 minutes**

Cooking time: **25 minutes**

Servings: **4**

Ingredients:

- 1 cup mozzarella, shredded
- 2 tablespoons olive oil
- 2 shallots, chopped

- 1 pound chicken breast, skinless, boneless and roughly cubed
- Salt and black pepper to the taste
- 1 cup carrots, sliced
- 1 teaspoon sweet paprika
- ¼ teaspoon onion powder
- ¼ teaspoon garlic powder
- ½ cup chicken stock
- 1 tablespoon chives, chopped

Directions:

In a saucepan, heat the oil on medium temperature, add the shallots, and cook for two minutes. Then add the carrots, chili powder garlic powder and onion Stir and cook for another 3 minutes. Add the meat and cook it for another 5 minutes. Then add the broth, then sprinkle the cheese, and cook for another 15 minutes. Sprinkle the chives over and divide the mixture among dishes and then serve.

Nutrition: calories 200, fat 4.5, fiber 3.5, carbs 8.5, protein 10

Beef Salad

Preparation time: **10 minutes**
Cooking time: **25 minutes**
Servings: **4**

Ingredients:

- 1 tablespoon lime juice
- 2 spring onions, chopped
- 2 shallots, chopped
- 2 garlic cloves, minced
- 2 tablespoons avocado oil
- 1 pound beef meat, ground
- 1 avocado, peeled, pitted and cubed
- 1 cup cherry tomatoes, halved
- 1 cup baby spinach
- A pinch of salt and black pepper
- ½ teaspoon hot paprika
- ¼ teaspoon chili powder
- 1 tablespoon cilantro, chopped
- 1 tablespoon chives, chopped

Directions:

In a pan, heat the oil at medium-low heat. Add garlic, shallots and spring onions. Stir and cook for 5 minutes. Add the meat and cook for 5 minutes longer. Add the remaining ingredients, mix gently cook on moderate heat for about 10 minutes, then divide into bowls, and serve at lunchtime.

Nutrition: calories 340, fat 30, fiber 5, carbs 3, protein 32

Green Beans Salad

Preparation time: **10 minutes**
Cooking time: **15 minutes**
Servings: **4**

Ingredients:

- 1 pound green beans, trimmed and halved
- 1 tablespoon olive oil
- 2 garlic cloves, minced
- 2 spring onions, chopped
- ½ cup tomato passata
- A pinch of salt and black pepper
- 1 cup cherry tomatoes, halved
- 1 cup baby spinach
- 1 tablespoon lime juice
- 1 tablespoon balsamic vinegar
- ½ teaspoon cumin, ground

Directions:

In a saucepan, heat the oil at medium-low heat. Add the garlic and spring onions. Stir and cook for two minutes. Then add the beans, and other ingredients, and bring to a boil at medium-low heat. Cook for 12 minutes, then divide into bowls, and serve for lunch.

Nutrition: calories 320, fat 8, fiber 4, carbs 3, protein 10

Beef Meatballs

Preparation time: **10 minutes**
Cooking time: **14 minutes**

Servings: **6**

Ingredients:

- 2 pounds beef, ground
- 2 eggs, whisked
- 1 tablespoon garlic, minced
- 1 tablespoon sweet paprika
- 1 tablespoon cilantro, chopped
- 2 tablespoons almond meal
- 2 shallots, chopped
- 2 tablespoons olive oil

Directions:

In a bowl mix the beef with the garlic and paprika, and the other ingredients, excluding the oil. Stir and form medium meatballs of the mix. In a skillet, heat the oil on medium heat. Add the meatballs and cook for about 6-7 minutes each side. Then, divide the meatballs between plates, and serve for lunch.

Nutrition: calories 180, fat 8, fiber 1, carbs 4, protein 20

Chicken Meatballs and Sauce

Preparation time: **10 minutes**
Cooking time: **30 minutes**
Servings: **4**

Ingredients:

For the sauce:

- 2 shallots, chopped
- 1 tablespoon olive oil
- 1 cup tomato passata
- 4 garlic cloves, minced
- 1 tablespoon balsamic vinegar

For the meatballs:

- 2 pounds chicken meat, skinless, boneless and ground
- 2 eggs, whisked
- 2 spring onions, chopped
- 2 tablespoons almond flour
- 2 tablespoons cilantro, chopped

Directions:

In a bowl, combine the meat with the eggs, spring onions, flour and the cilantro, stir well and shape medium meatballs out of this mix. In a skillet, heat the oil on medium temperature, add the meatballs and cook them for 2 minutes each side, then transfer them to a dish. In the same pan, heat at medium-low heat, add the shallots and garlic Stir and cook until the garlic is tender for five minutes. Add the passata and vinegar. Stir and cook the sauce for 3 minutes. Add the meatballs and cook for an additional 15 minutes then divide the mixture into bowls, and serve as lunch.

Nutrition: calories 340, fat 12.6, fiber 6.4, carbs 7, protein 12.5

Shrimp and Zucchini Pan

Preparation time: **5 minutes**
Cooking time: **8 minutes**
Servings: **4**

Ingredients:

- 1 tablespoon olive oil
- 1 pound shrimp, peeled and deveined
- 1 cup zucchinis, sliced
- 2 shallots, chopped
- 1 tablespoon garlic, minced
- 1 tablespoon red chili flakes
- A pinch of salt and black pepper
- 1 tablespoon basil, chopped

Directions:

Prepare a pan using the oil and the ghee over medium-high heat. Add the shallots and garlic, stir and cook for two minutes. Add the zucchinis, shrimp as well as the other ingredients. Cook for an additional 6 minutes then divide the dish into plates and serve with lunch.

Nutrition: calories 176, fat 5.5, fiber 0.4, carbs 4.2, protein 26.5

Avocado and Zucchini Salad

Preparation time: **10 minutes**
Cooking time: **0 minutes**
Servings: **4**

Ingredients:

- 1 cup arugula
- 1 avocado, peeled, pitted and cut into wedges
- 3 cups zucchini noodles
- ½ cup mozzarella, shredded
- 1 tablespoon avocado oil
- 1 tablespoon balsamic vinegar
- 1 cup cherry tomatoes, halved
- A pinch of salt and black pepper

Directions:

In a bowl for salad mix the zucchini noodles with the arugula as well as the other ingredients. Toss and serve as a lunch.

Nutrition: calories 141, fat 11.1, fiber 5.1, carbs 9.5, protein 3.6

Dill Salmon Salad

Preparation time: **10 minutes**
Cooking time: **0 minutes**
Servings: **2**

Ingredients:

- ½ cup green onion, chopped
- 2 smoked salmon fillets, boneless, skinless and roughly shredded
- 2 tablespoons dill, chopped
- 1 avocado, peeled, pitted and roughly cubed
- ½ tablespoons balsamic vinegar
- 1 tablespoon olive oil
- Salt and black pepper to the taste
- 2 tablespoons prepared horseradish

Directions:

In a bowl, combine the salmon with the green onion and the other ingredients, toss and serve for lunch.

Nutrition: calories 467, fat 38.1, fiber 8.3, carbs 14.9, protein 4.3

Balsamic Steaks

Preparation time: **10 minutes**
Cooking time: **15 minutes**
Servings: **4**

Ingredients:

1 pound beef steaks, cut into 4 sliced

2 tablespoons olive oil

Salt and black pepper to the taste

¼ cup balsamic vinegar

2 garlic cloves, minced

1 teaspoon red pepper flakes

1 teaspoon garlic powder

2 shallots, chopped

1 tablespoon chives, chopped

Directions:

Prepare a pan using the oil at medium-low temperature, then add the shallots, garlic as well as pepper flakes and garlic powder. Stir, and cook for five minutes. Add the steaks along with all the ingredients and cook for 5 minutes each side. Divide them into plates and serve.

Nutrition: calories 435, fat 23, fiber 7, carbs 10, protein 35

Turkey and Endives Salad

Preparation time: **10 minutes**
Cooking time: **0 minutes**
Servings: **4**

Ingredients:

1 turkey breast, skinless, boneless, cooked and cut into strips

2 tablespoons avocado oil

2 endives, shredded

1 cup cherry tomatoes, halved

2 tablespoons lime juice

2 tablespoons balsamic vinegar

2 tablespoons chives, chopped

Salt and black pepper to the taste

Directions:

In a bowl make a mix of the turkey with the endives as well as the other ingredients. Mix and serve as a lunch.

Nutrition: calories 200, fat 10, fiber 1.54, carbs 3, protein 7

Avocado Salad

Preparation time: **5 minutes**
Cooking time: **0 minutes**
Servings: **2**

Ingredients:
2 big avocados, pitted, peeled and cut into wedges
1 tablespoon olive oil
1 cup kalamata olives, pitted and halved
1 cup cucumber, sliced
1 tablespoon lime juice
A pinch of salt and black pepper

Directions: In a salad bowl, combine the avocados with the olives and the other ingredients, toss and serve cold for lunch.

Nutrition: calories 230, fat 13.4, fiber 12, carbs 5, protein 6.7

Chicken Stew

Preparation time: **10 minutes**
Cooking time: **20 minutes**
Servings: **4**

Ingredients:
1 pound chicken breast, skinless, boneless and cubed
1 cup chicken stock
½ cup tomato passata
1 red onion, chopped

1 tablespoon avocado oil
1 red bell pepper, cubed
1 shallot, chopped
A pinch of salt and black pepper
2 garlic cloves, minced
1 cup cherry tomatoes, halved
1 tablespoon cilantro, chopped

Directions:

In a pan, heat the oil on medium temperature, add the garlic and shallot and cook for two minutes. Add the meat and cook it for three minutes. Add the stock and other ingredients, bring it to the point of simmering and cook on medium heat for about 15 minutes while stirring from the time. Divide the stew into bowls, and serve as a lunch.

Nutrition: calories 357, fat 23, fiber 5, carbs 6.3, protein 26

Beef and Radish Stew

Preparation time: **10 minutes**
Cooking time: **32 minutes**
Servings: **4**

Ingredients:
1 pound beef stew meat, cubed
2 shallots, chopped
2 tablespoons olive oil
2 garlic cloves, minced
1 cup radishes, cubed
1 cup black olives, pitted and halved
1 cup tomato passata
1 cup beef stock
½ teaspoon rosemary, dried
½ teaspoon oregano, dried
1 tablespoon parsley, chopped
A pinch of salt and black pepper

Directions:

In a large pot, heat the oil at medium-high heat. Add the shallot and garlic and sauté for two minutes. Add the meat and cook for another 5 minutes. Add the olives, radishes and the rest of the ingredients. Bring to a boil and cook at medium-low temperature for another 25 minutes with a stirring often. Divide the stew among dishes and enjoy.

Nutrition: calories 456, fat 32, fiber 2, carbs 6, protein 30

Salmon Bowls

Preparation time: **10 minutes**
Cooking time: **15 minutes**
Servings: **4**

Ingredients:

1 pound salmon fillets, boneless, skinless and roughly cubed

1 cup chicken stock

2 spring onions, chopped

1 tablespoon olive oil

1 cup kalamata olives, pitted and halved

1 avocado, pitted, peeled and roughly cubed

1 cup baby spinach

A pinch of salt and black pepper

¼ cup cilantro, chopped

1 tablespoon basil, chopped

1 teaspoon lime juice

Directions:

In a pan, heat the oil on medium heat. Add the spring onions and salmon, mix gently then cook for 5 mins. Add the olives and other ingredients and cook on medium temperature for another 10 minutes. Divide the mixture into bowls and serve it for lunch.

Nutrition: calories 254, fat 17, fiber 1.9, carbs 6.1, protein 20

Beef and Kale pan

Preparation time: **10 minutes**
Cooking time: **20 minutes**
Servings: **4**

Ingredients:

1 pound beef stew meat, cubed

1 red onion, chopped

1 tablespoon olive oil

2 garlic cloves, minced

1 cup kale, torn

1 cup beef stock

1 teaspoon chili powder

½ teaspoon sweet paprika

1 teaspoon rosemary, dried

1 tablespoon cilantro, chopped

A pinch of salt and black pepper

Directions:

Prepare a pan using the oil at medium-high heat. Add the garlic and the onion. Stir and cook for two minutes. Add the meat, and cook in 5 mins. Add the other ingredients, cook to an unbeatable simmer, then cook on moderate heat for 13 minutes more. Divide the mix among plates, and serve with lunch.

Nutrition: calories 160, fat 10, fiber 3, carbs 1, protein 12

Cheesy Pork Casserole

Preparation time: **10 minutes**
Cooking time: **40 minutes**
Servings: **4**

Ingredients:

1 cup cheddar cheese, grated

2 eggs, whisked

1 pound pork loin, cubed

2 tablespoons avocado oil

2 shallots, chopped

A pinch of salt and black pepper

3 garlic cloves, minced

1 cup red bell peppers, cut into strips

¼ cup heavy cream

1 tablespoon chives, chopped

½ teaspoon cumin, ground

Directions:

Prepare a pan using the oil on medium heat. Add the shallots and garlic, and cook for 2 minutes. Then add the bell peppers and the meat, mix well and cook for an additional 5 minutes. Mix the salt, cumin and pepper, toss, and then remove the pan from the fire. In a bowl, mix the eggs with the cream and the cheese, whisk and pour over the pork mix. Sprinkle the chives over the top, place the pan into the oven and bake at 350 degree F in 30 mins. Divide the mixture among plates and serve it for lunch.

Nutrition: calories 455, fat 34, fiber 3, carbs 3, protein 33

Thyme Chicken Mix

Preparation time: **10 minutes**
Cooking time: **20 minutes**
Servings: **4**

Ingredients:

1 pound chicken breast, skinless, boneless and cut into strips

1 tablespoon olive oil

2 spring onions, chopped

1 cup baby spinach

1 tablespoon thyme, chopped

½ cup tomato passata

A pinch of salt and black pepper

Directions:

Heat up a pan with the oil over medium heat, add the spring onions and the meat and brown for 5 minutes. Add the remaining ingredients and bring to the point of simmering and cook on moderate heat for about 15 minutes while stirring from time

to time. Divide the mixture in bowls and then serve.

Nutrition: calories 380, fat 40, fiber 5, carbs 1, protein 17

Chicken Soup

Preparation time: **10 minutes**
Cooking time: **8 hours**
Servings: **4**

Ingredients:

1 pound chicken breast, skinless, boneless and cubed

2 tablespoons olive oil

2 shallots, chopped

2 zucchinis, sliced

1 quart chicken stock

Juice from 1 lime

2 chili peppers chopped

2 tablespoons cilantro, chopped

Directions:

In a slow cooker, mix the meat, oil, shallots, and other ingredients. Place the lid in and cook at low until 8 hours. Divide the soup into bowls and serve.

Nutrition: calories 300, fat 5, fiber 6, carbs 3, protein 26

Zucchini Soup

Preparation time: **10 minutes**
Cooking time: **22 minutes**
Servings: **4**

Ingredients:

1 quart chicken stock

1 pound zucchinis, roughly cubed

1 tablespoon avocado oil

2 shallots, chopped

½ cup heavy cream

1 tablespoon dill, chopped

A pinch of salt and black pepper

1 teaspoon ginger powder

Juice of 1 lime

Directions:

In a large pot, heat the oil at medium-low temperature, add the shallots and stir-fry for two minutes. Add the zucchinis and stock, salt, pepper, and the ginger powder mix, bring the soup to a boil to cook the soup for about 15 mins. Add the lime and cream juice, Blend the soup using an immersion blender. Warm it up on medium temperature for another 5 minutes. Divide the soup into bowls, add the dill over top and serve with lunch.

Nutrition: calories 450, fat 34, fiber 4, carbs 8, protein 12

Lime Turkey Soup

Preparation time: **10 minutes**

Cooking time: **30 minutes**

Servings: **4**

Ingredients:

1 pound turkey breast, skinless, boneless and cubed

2 shallots, chopped

2 tablespoons olive oil

2 garlic cloves, minced

2 tomatoes, cubed

1 jalapeno pepper, chopped

6 cups chicken stock

A pinch of salt and black pepper

1 red bell pepper, chopped

2 tablespoons parsley, chopped

1 tablespoon lime juice

Directions:

In a large pot, heat the oil on medium heat. Add the shallots and garlic, and cook for 2 minutes. Add the tomatoes, meat and other ingredients, except for the parsley. Bring to a boil, then cook on the medium heat for around 28 minutes. Pour this soup in bowls and sprinkle the parsley over and serve.

Nutrition: calories 287, fat 14, fiber 2, carbs 7, protein 25

Beef Curry

Preparation time: **10 minutes**

Cooking time: **45 minutes**

Servings: **4**

Ingredients:

2 tablespoons olive oil

1 pound beef stew meat, cubed

2 shallots, chopped

1 cup beef stock

2 cups coconut milk

1 tablespoon lime juice

3 garlic cloves, minced

1 tablespoon cilantro, chopped

1 tablespoon ginger, grated

2 tablespoons red curry paste

1 teaspoon turmeric, ground

1 teaspoon cumin, ground

Directions:

In a large pot, heat the oil at medium high heat. Add garlic, shallots and ginger, stir and cook for 5 minutes. Add the meat, and the curry paste, mix well and cook for 5 minutes. Add the stock and the additional ingredients. Bring it to the point of simmering and cook on medium-high heat for approximately 35 minutes. Stir regularly. Divide the curry into bowls and serve for lunch.

Nutrition: calories 430, fat 22, fiber 4, carbs 7, protein 53

Lunch Spinach Rolls

Preparation time: **20 minutes**

Cooking time: **15 minutes**

Servings: **16**

Ingredients:

6 tablespoons coconut flour

½ cup almond flour

2 and ½ cups mozzarella cheese, shredded

2 eggs

A pinch of salt

For the filling:

4 ounces cream cheese

6 ounces spinach, torn

A drizzle of avocado oil

A pinch of salt

¼ cup parmesan, grated

Mayonnaise for serving

Directions:

Heat up a pan with the oil over medium heat, add spinach and cook for 2 minutes. Add parmesan, a pinch of salt and cream cheese, stir well, take off heat and leave aside for now. Put mozzarella cheese in a heat proof bowl and microwave for 30 seconds. Add eggs, salt, coconut and almond flour and stir everything. Place dough on a lined cutting board, place a parchment paper on top and flatten dough with a rolling pin. Divide dough into 16 rectangles, spread spinach mix on each and roll them into cigar shapes. Place all rolls on a lined baking sheet, introduce in the oven at 350 degrees F and bake for 15 minutes. Leave rolls to cool down for a few minutes before serving them with some mayo on top. Enjoy!

Nutrition: calories 500, fat 65, fiber 4, carbs 14, protein 32

Delicious Steak Bowl

Preparation time: **15 minutes**

Cooking time: **8 minutes**

Servings: **4**

Ingredients:

16 ounces skirt steak

4 ounces pepper jack cheese, shredded

1 cup sour cream

Salt and black pepper to the taste

1 handful cilantro, chopped

A splash of chipotle adobo sauce

For the guacamole:

¼ cup red onion, chopped

2 avocados, pitted and peeled

Juice from 1 lime

1 tablespoon olive oil

6 cherry tomatoes, chopped

1 garlic clove, minced

1 tablespoon cilantro, chopped

Salt and black pepper to the taste

Directions:

Put avocados in a bowl and mash with a fork. Add tomatoes, red onion, garlic, salt and pepper and stir well. Add olive oil, lime juice and 1 tablespoon cilantro, stir again very well and leave aside for now. Heat up a pan over high heat, add steak, season with salt and pepper, cook for 4 minutes on each side, transfer to a cutting board, leave aside to cool down a bit and cut in thin strips. Divide steak into 4 bowls, add cheese, sour cream and guacamole on top and serve with a splash of chipotle adobo sauce.

Enjoy!

Nutrition: calories 600, fat 50, fiber 6, carbs 5, protein 30

Meatballs And Pilaf

Preparation time: **10 minutes**

Cooking time: **30 minutes**

Servings: **4**

Ingredients:

12 ounces cauliflower florets

Salt and black pepper to the taste

1 egg

1 pound lamb, ground

1 teaspoon fennel seed

1 teaspoon paprika

1 teaspoon garlic powder

1 small yellow onion, chopped

2 garlic cloves, minced

2 tablespoons coconut oil

1 bunch mint, chopped

1 tablespoon lemon zest

4 ounces goat cheese, crumbled

Directions:

Put cauliflower florets in your food processor, add salt and pulse well. Grease a pan with some of the coconut oil, heat up over medium heat, add cauliflower rice, cook for 8 minutes, season with salt and pepper to the taste, take off heat and keep warm. In a bowl, mix lamb with salt, pepper, egg, paprika, garlic powder and fennel seed and stir very well. Shape 12 meatballs and place them on a plate for now. Heat up a pan with the coconut oil over medium heat, add onion, stir and cook for 6 minutes. Add garlic, stir and cook for 1 minute. Add meatballs, cook them well on all sides and take off heat. Divide cauliflower rice on plates, add meatballs and onion mix on top, sprinkle mint, lemon zest and goat cheese at the end and serve. Enjoy!

Nutrition: calories 470, fat 43, fiber 5, carbs 4, protein 26

Delicious Broccoli Soup

Preparation time: **10 minutes**

Cooking time: **30 minutes**

Servings: **4**

Ingredients:

1 white onion, chopped

1 tablespoon ghee

2 cups veggie stock

Salt and black pepper to the taste

2 cups water

2 garlic cloves, minced

1 cup heavy cream

8 ounces cheddar cheese, grated

12 ounces broccoli florets

½ teaspoon paprika

Directions:

Heat up a pot with the ghee over medium heat, add onion and garlic, stir and cook for 5 minutes. Add stock, cream, water, salt, pepper and paprika, stir and bring to a boil. Add broccoli, stir and simmer soup for 25 minutes. Transfer to your food processor and blend well. Add cheese and blend again. Divide into soup bowls and serve hot. Enjoy!

Nutrition: calories 350, fat 34, fiber 7, carbs 7, protein 11

Lunch Green Beans Salad

Preparation time: **10 minutes**

Cooking time: **5 minutes**

Servings: **8**

Ingredients:

2 tablespoons white wine vinegar

1 and ½ tablespoons mustard

Salt and black pepper to the taste

2 pounds green beans

1/3 cup extra virgin olive oil

1 and ½ cups fennel, thinly sliced

4 ounces goat cheese, crumbled

¾ cup walnuts, toasted and chopped

Directions:

Put water in a pot, add some salt and bring to a boil over medium high heat. Add green beans, cook for 5 minutes and transfer them to a bowl filled with ice water. Drain green beans well and put them in a salad bowl. Add walnuts, fennel and goat cheese and toss gently. In a bowl, mix vinegar with mustard, salt, pepper and oil and whisk well. Pour this over salad, toss to coat well and serve for lunch. Enjoy!

Nutrition: calories 200, fat 14, fiber 4, carbs 5,

protein 6

Pumpkin Soup

Preparation time: **10 minutes**
Cooking time: **20 minutes**
Servings: **6**

Ingredients:
½ cup yellow onion, chopped
2 tablespoons olive oil
1 tablespoon chipotles in adobo sauce
1 garlic clove, minced
1 teaspoon cumin, ground
1 teaspoon coriander, ground
A pinch of allspice
2 cups pumpkin puree
Salt and black pepper to the taste
32 ounces chicken stock
½ cup heavy cream
2 teaspoons vinegar
2 teaspoons stevia

Directions:
Heat up a pot with the oil over medium heat, add onions and garlic, stir and cook for 4 minutes. Add stevia, cumin, coriander, chipotles and cumin, stir and cook for 2 minutes. Add stock and pumpkin puree, stir and cook for 5 minutes. Blend soup well using an immersion blender and then mix with salt, pepper, heavy cream and vinegar. Stir, cook for 5 minutes more and divide into bowls. Serve right away. Enjoy!

Nutrition: calories 140, fat 12, fiber 3, carbs 6, protein 2

Delicious Green Beans Casserole

Preparation time: **10 minutes**
Cooking time: **35 minutes**
Servings: **8**

Ingredients:
1 pound green beans, halved
Salt and black pepper to the taste
½ cup almond flour
2 tablespoons ghee
8 ounces mushrooms, chopped
4 ounces onion, chopped
2 shallots, chopped
3 garlic cloves, minced
½ cup chicken stock
½ cup heavy cream
¼ cup parmesan, grated
Avocado oil for frying

Directions:
Put some water in a pot, add salt, bring to a boil over medium high heat, add green beans, cook for 5 minutes, transfer to a bowl filled with ice water, cool down, drain well and leave aside for now. In a bowl, mix shallots with onions, almond flour, salt and pepper and toss to coat. Heat up a pan with some avocado oil over medium high heat, add onions and shallots mix, fry until they are golden. Transfer to paper towels and drain grease. Heat up the same pan over medium heat, add ghee and melt it. Add garlic and mushrooms, stir and cook for 5 minutes. Add stock and heavy cream, stir, bring to a boil and simmer until it thickens. Add parmesan and green beans, toss to coat and take off heat. Transfer this mix to a baking dish, sprinkle crispy onions mix all over, introduce in the oven at 400 degrees F and bake for 15 minutes. Serve warm. Enjoy!

Nutrition: calories 155, fat, 11, fiber 6, carbs 8, protein 5

Simple Lunch Apple Salad

Preparation time: **10 minutes**
Cooking time: **0 minutes**
Servings: **4**

Ingredients:

2 cups broccoli florets, roughly chopped

2 ounces pecans, chopped

1 apple, cored and grated

1 green onion stalk, finely chopped

Salt and black pepper to the taste

2 teaspoons poppy seeds

1 teaspoon apple cider vinegar

¼ cup mayonnaise

½ teaspoon lemon juice

¼ cup sour cream

Directions:

In a salad bowl, mix apple with broccoli, green onion and pecans and stir. Add poppy seeds, salt and pepper and toss gently. In a bowl, mix mayo with sour cream, vinegar and lemon juice and whisk well. Pour this over salad, toss to coat well and serve cold for lunch! Enjoy!

Nutrition: calories 250, fat 23, fiber 4, carbs 4, protein 5

Brussels Sprouts Gratin

Preparation time: **10 minutes**

Cooking time: **35 minutes**

Servings: **4**

Ingredients:

2 ounces onions, chopped

1 teaspoon garlic, minced

6 ounces Brussels sprouts, chopped

2 tablespoons ghee

1 tablespoon coconut aminos

Salt and black pepper to the taste

½ teaspoon liquid smoke

For the sauce:

2.5 ounces cheddar cheese, grated

A pinch of black pepper

1 tablespoon ghee

½ cup heavy cream

¼ teaspoon turmeric

¼ teaspoon paprika

A pinch of xanthan gum

For the pork crust:

3 tablespoons parmesan

0.5 ounces pork rinds

½ teaspoon sweet paprika

Directions:

Heat up a pan with 2 tablespoons ghee over high heat, add Brussels sprouts, salt and pepper, stir and cook for 3 minutes. Add garlic and onion, stir and cook for 3 minutes more. Add liquid smoke and coconut aminos, stir, take off heat and leave aside for now. Heat up another pan with 1 tablespoon ghee over medium heat, add heavy cream and stir. Add cheese, black pepper, turmeric, paprika and xanthan gum, stir and cook until it thickens again. Add Brussels sprouts mix, toss to coat and divide into ramekins. In your food processor, mix parmesan with pork rinds and ½ teaspoon paprika and pulse well. Divide these crumbs on top of Brussels sprouts mix, introduce ramekins in the oven at 375 degrees F and bake for 20 minutes. Serve right away. Enjoy!

Nutrition: calories 300, fat 20, fiber 6, carbs 5, protein 10

Simple Asparagus Lunch

Preparation time: **10 minutes**

Cooking time: **10 minutes**

Servings: **4**

Ingredients:

2 egg yolks

Salt and black pepper to the taste

¼ cup ghee

1 tablespoon lemon juice

A pinch of cayenne pepper

40 asparagus spears

Directions:

In a bowl, whisk egg yolks very well. Transfer this to a small pan over low heat. Add lemon juice and whisk well. Add ghee and whisk until it melts. Add salt, pepper and cayenne pepper and whisk again well. Meanwhile, heat up a pan over medium high heat, add asparagus spears and fry them for 5 minutes. Divide asparagus on plates, drizzle the sauce you've made on top and serve. Enjoy!

Nutrition: calories 150, fat 13, fiber 6, carbs 2, protein 3

Simple Shrimp Pasta

Preparation time: **10 minutes**
Cooking time: **10 minutes**
Servings: **4**

Ingredients:

12 ounces angel hair noodles

2 tablespoons olive oil

Salt and black pepper to the taste

2 tablespoons ghee

4 garlic cloves, minced

1 pound shrimp, raw, peeled and deveined

Juice from ½ lemon

½ teaspoon paprika

A handful basil, chopped

Directions:

Put water in a pot, add some salt, bring to a bo, then add noodles. Cook for two minutes, then drain and transfer to a heated pan. Toast the noodles for a couple of seconds, remove from heat and set to cool. Prepare a pan using the olive oil and ghee on medium heat. Add garlic, stir and cook for about 1 minute. Add the shrimp and lemon juice, and take 3 minutes to cook per side. Mix noodles with salt, pepper, and paprika. Stir to combine, then divide into bowls serving with the chopped basil over the top. Enjoy!

Nutrition: calories 300, fat 20, fiber 6, carbs 3, protein 30

Incredible Mexican Casserole

Preparation time: **10 minutes**
Cooking time: **35 minutes**

Servings: **6**

Ingredients:

2 chipotle peppers, chopped

2 jalapenos, chopped

1 tablespoon olive oil

¼ cup heavy cream

1 small white onion, chopped

Salt and black pepper to the taste

1 pound chicken thighs, skinless, boneless and chopped

1 cup red enchilada sauce

4 ounces cream cheese

Cooking spray

1 cup pepper jack cheese, shredded

2 tablespoons cilantro, chopped

2 tortillas

Directions:

Prepare a pan using the oil at medium-high heat. Add chipotle and jalapeno peppers. stir and cook for a few seconds. Add the onion, stir to cook 5 mins. Add heavy cream and cream cheese stir until the cheese is melted. Add chicken, salt, pepper and enchilada sauce. Stir thoroughly and then turn off the heat. Clean a baking dish by spraying cooking oil, put tortillas in the bottom then spread the chicken mix over and top with shredded cheese. Cover with foil, bake to 350° F then bake it for about 15 minutes. Remove the foil from the oven and bake for an additional 15 minutes. Sprinkle with cilantro and serve. Enjoy!

Nutrition: calories 240, fat 12, fiber 5, carbs 5, protein 20

Delicious Asian Lunch Salad

Preparation time: **10 minutes**
Cooking time: **15 minutes**
Servings: **4**

Ingredients:

1 pound beef, ground

1 tablespoon sriracha

2 tablespoons coconut aminos

2 garlic cloves, minced

10 ounces cole slaw mix

2 tablespoon sesame seed oil

Salt and black pepper to the taste

1 teaspoon apple cider vinegar

1 teaspoon sesame seeds

1 green onion stalk, chopped

Directions:

In a pan, heat the oil on medium heat. Add garlic and cook for one minute. Add the beef, stir until cooked for 10 minutes. Mix in cole slaw, toss until coated and cook for 1 minute. Mix in vinegar, sriracha and vinegar, coconut aminos, salt and pepper, mix and cook for another 4 minutes. Include sesame seeds and green onions. toss to coat, divide into bowls and serve for lunch. Enjoy!

Nutrition: calories 350, fat 23, fiber 6, carbs 3, protein 20

Simple Buffalo Wings

Preparation time: **10 minutes**

Cooking time: **20 minutes**

Servings: **2**

Ingredients:

2 tablespoons ghee

6 chicken wings, cut in halves

Salt and black pepper to the taste

A pinch of garlic powder

½ cup hot sauce

A pinch of cayenne pepper

½ teaspoon sweet paprika

Directions:

In a bowl mix the chicken parts with the half hot sauce along with salt and pepper. Combine thoroughly to coat. Place chicken pieces in a baking dish lined with baking parchment then place in the oven and bake for 8 minutes. Turn chicken pieces over and then broil for 8 minutes further. Then, heat a pan with the ghee at medium-high temperature. Add the remaining hot sauce and salt, cayenne, pepper and paprika. Mix and cook for about a few minutes. Transfer broiled chicken pieces to a bowl, add ghee and hot sauce mix over them and toss to coat well. Serve them right away! Enjoy!

Nutrition: calories 500, fat 45, fiber 12, carbs 1, protein 45

Amazing Bacon And Mushrooms Skewers

Preparation time: **10 minutes**

Cooking time: **20 minutes**

Servings: **6**

Ingredients:

1 pound mushroom caps

6 bacon strips

Salt and black pepper to the taste

½ teaspoon sweet paprika

Some sweet mesquite

Directions:

Season mushrooms with salt, pepper, and paprika. Spread bacon strips onto the skewer's end. Use a mushroom cap to braid bacon over it. Repeat until you have bacon and a mushroom. Repeat the process with the rest of the bacon strips and mushrooms. Add sweet mesquite to the mix, place all skewers on a preheated cooking grills on medium-high temperature, cook for 10 minutes before flipping and cook for another 10 minutes. Serve the skewers on plates as a lunch, with salad! Enjoy!

Nutrition: calories 110, fat 7, fiber 4, carbs 2, protein 10

Simple Tomato Soup

Preparation time: **10 minutes**

Cooking time: **5 minutes**

Servings: **4**

Ingredients:

1 quart canned tomato soup

4 tablespoons ghee

¼ cup olive oil

¼ cup red hot sauce

2 tablespoons apple cider vinegar

Salt and black pepper to the taste

1 teaspoon oregano, dried

2 teaspoon turmeric, ground

8 bacon strips, cooked and crumbled

A handful green onions, chopped

A handful basil leaves, chopped

Directions:

Place tomato soup in the pot and cook on medium temperature. Mix olive oil, and ghee, vinegar, hot sauce, salt, pepper, oregano and turmeric, stir and cook until 5 mins. Remove from the heat, divide the soup into bowls, and top with bacon pieces, green onions and basil. Enjoy!

Nutrition: calories 400, fat 34, fiber 7, carbs 10, protein 12

Bacon Wrapped Sausages

Preparation time: **10 minutes**

Cooking time: **30 minutes**

Servings: **4**

Ingredients:

8 bacon strips

8 sausages

16 pepper jack cheese slices

Salt and black pepper to the taste

A pinch of garlic powder

½ teaspoon sweet paprika

1 pinch of onion powder

Directions:

Heat up your kitchen grill over medium heat, add

sausages, cook for a few minutes on each side, transfer to a plate and leave them aside for a few minutes to cool down. Cut a slit in the middle of each sausage to create pockets, stuff each with 2 cheese slices and season with salt, pepper, paprika, onion and garlic powder. Wrap each stuffed sausage in a bacon strip, secure with toothpicks, place on a lined baking sheet, introduce in the oven at 400 degrees F and bake for 15 minutes. Serve hot for lunch! Enjoy!

Nutrition: calories 500, fat 37, fiber 12, carbs 4, protein 40

Lunch Lobster Bisque

Preparation time: **10 minutes**

Cooking time: **1 hour**

Servings: **4**

Ingredients:

4 garlic cloves, minced

1 small red onion, chopped

24 ounces lobster chunks, pre-cooked

Salt and black pepper to the taste

½ cup tomato paste

2 carrots, finely chopped

4 celery stalks, chopped

1 quart seafood stock

1 tablespoon olive oil

1 cup heavy cream

3 bay leaves

1 teaspoon thyme, dried

1 teaspoon peppercorns

1 teaspoon paprika

1 teaspoon xantham gum

A handful parsley, chopped

1 tablespoon lemon juice

Directions:

In a large pot, heat the oil on medium temperature, add the onion, stir, and cook for four minutes. Add garlic stir, cook for another minute. Add celery and carrots, Stir and cook for one minute. Mix tomato paste as well as stock and stir it all in. Include bay leaf, salt peppercorns, peppercorns, thyme, paprika and xantham gum. Stir and simmer on moderate heat for one hour. Take out bay leaves, add cream and simmer. Blend with an immersion blender. Add lobster pieces and simmer for few more minutes. Mix in lemon juice, mix to combine, then divide into bowls and add parsley to the top. Enjoy!

Nutrition: calories 200, fat 12, fiber 7, carbs 6, protein 12

Simple Halloumi Salad

Preparation time: **10 minutes**
Cooking time: **10 minutes**
Servings: **1**

Ingredients:

3 ounces halloumi cheese, sliced

1 cucumber, sliced

1 ounce walnuts, chopped

A drizzle of olive oil

A handful baby arugula

5 cherry tomatoes, halved

A splash of balsamic vinegar

Salt and black pepper to the taste

Directions:

Heat up your kitchen grill over medium high heat, add halloumi pieces, grill them for 5 minutes on each side and transfer to a plate. In a bowl mix tomatoes, walnuts, cucumber, and arugula. Place halloumi pieces over the top, season everything with salt and pepper, drizzle vinegar and oil on top in a bowl, mix to coat, and serve. Enjoy!

Nutrition: calories 450, fat 43, fiber 5, carbs 4, protein 21

Lunch Stew

Preparation time: **10 minutes**
Cooking time: 3 hours and 30 minutes

Servings: **6**

Ingredients:

8 tomatoes, chopped

5 pounds beef shanks

3 carrots, chopped

8 garlic cloves, minced

2 onions, chopped

2 cups water

1 quart chicken stock

¼ cup tomato sauce

Salt and black pepper to the taste

2 tablespoons apple cider vinegar

3 bay leaves

3 teaspoons red pepper, crushed

2 teaspoons parsley, dried

2 teaspoons basil, dried

2 teaspoons garlic powder

2 teaspoons onion powder

A pinch of cayenne pepper

Directions:

Cook a pot on medium heat. Add onions, carrots, and garlic, Stir and cook for a couple of minutes. Heat up a pan over medium heat, add beef shank, brown for a few minutes on each side and take off heat. Put the carrots in the stock along with the water and vinegar, and stir. Add tomatoes, tomato sauce, salt, pepper, cayenne pepper crushed pepper, bay leaves, parsley, basil, onion powder and garlic powder. Mix everything. Add the beef shanks, cover pot with water, reduce heat to a simmer to cook 3 hours. Discard bay leaves, divide into bowls and serve. Enjoy!

Nutrition: calories 500, fat 22, fiber 4, carbs 6, protein 56

Chicken And Shrimp

Preparation time: **10 minutes**
Cooking time: **20 minutes**
Servings: **2**

Ingredients:

20 shrimp, raw, peeled and deveined

2 chicken breasts, boneless and skinless

2 handfuls spinach leaves

½ pound mushrooms, roughly chopped

Salt and black pepper to the taste

¼ cup mayonnaise

2 tablespoons sriracha

2 teaspoons lime juice

1 tablespoon coconut oil

½ teaspoon red pepper, crushed

1 teaspoon garlic powder

½ teaspoon paprika

¼ teaspoon xantham gum

1 green onion stalk, chopped

Directions:

In a pan, heat the oil on medium-high temperature, add the chicken breasts and season using salt, pepper, garlic powder and red pepper and cook for 8 minutes. Flip and cook for an additional 6 minutes. Add the mushrooms, salt and pepper, and cook for about 5 minutes. Heat up another pan over medium heat, add shrimp, sriracha, paprika, xantham and mayo, stir and cook until shrimp turn pink. Remove the pan from the heat. Add lime juice and mix everything. Divide the spinach onto plates, and divide between mushrooms and chicken. Top with shrimp mix. Garnish with green onions and serve. Enjoy!

Nutrition: calories 500, fat 34, fiber 10, carbs 3, protein 40

Green Soup

Preparation time: **10 minutes**

Cooking time: **13 minutes**

Servings: **6**

Ingredients:

1 cauliflower head, florets separated

1 white onion, finely chopped

1 bay leaf, crushed

2 garlic cloves, minced

5 ounces watercress

7 ounces spinach leaves

1 quart veggie stock

1 cup coconut milk

Salt and black pepper to the taste

¼ cup ghee

A handful parsley, for serving

Directions:

In a large pot, heat the ghee at medium high heat. Add onions and garlic. Stir and cook for four minutes. Add bay leaf and cauliflower to cook, stir and cook in 5 mins. Add the spinach and watercress, Stir to cook 3 mins. Add salt, stock and pepper. Stir and bring to an even boil. Stir in coconut milk remove from heat and blend with the aid of an immersion blender. Divide into bowls and serve now. Enjoy!

Nutrition: calories 230, fat 34, fiber 3, carbs 5, protein 7

Caprese Salad

Preparation time: **5 minutes**

Cooking time: **0 minutes**

Servings: **2**

Ingredients:

½ pound mozzarella cheese, sliced

1 tomato, sliced

Salt and black pepper to the taste

4 basil leaves, torn

1 tablespoon balsamic vinegar

1 tablespoon olive oil

Directions:

Alternate tomato and mozzarella slices on 2 plates. Sprinkle salt and pepper, drizzle vinegar and olive oil. Sprinkle basil leaves in the middle and serve. Enjoy!

Nutrition: calories 150, fat 12, fiber 5, carbs 6, protein 9

Salmon Soup

Preparation time: **10 minutes**
Cooking time: **25 minutes**
Servings: **4**

Ingredients:

4 leeks, trimmed and sliced

Salt and black pepper to the taste

2 tablespoons avocado oil

2 garlic cloves, minced

6 cups chicken stock

1 pound salmon, cut in small pieces

2 teaspoons thyme, dried

1 and ¾ cups coconut milk

Directions:

In a large pot, heat the oil on medium heat. Add garlic and leeks. Stir and cook in 5 mins. Add thyme and stock along with salt and pepper. Stir, and cook over 15 minutes. Add the coconut milk and salmon, Stir, then return to a simmer. Divide into bowls and serve now. Enjoy!

Nutrition: calories 270, fat 12, fiber 3, carbs 5, protein 32

Amazing Halibut Soup

Preparation time: **10 minutes**
Cooking time: **30 minutes**
Servings: **4**

Ingredients:

1 yellow onion, chopped

1 pound carrots, sliced

1 tablespoon coconut oil

Salt and black pepper to the taste

2 tablespoons ginger, minced

1 cup water

1 pound halibut, cut in medium chunks

12 cups chicken stock

Directions:

In a large pot, heat the oil on medium-high heat. Add the onions, stir and cook for about 6 minutes. Add carrots, ginger along with the stock and water and stir. Bring to a simmer, lower temperature, and allow to simmer for around 10 minutes. Blend soup with an immersion blender, then season with salt and pepper, and add pieces of halibut. Stir well and cook the soup for another 5 minutes. Divide soup into bowls and serve. Enjoy!

Nutrition: calories 140, fat 6, fiber 1, carbs 4, protein 14

Cheddar & Broccoli Soup

Ingredients for 4 servings

¾ cup heavy cream

1 onion, diced

1 tsp minced garlic

4 cups chopped broccoli

4 cups veggie broth

2 tbsp butter

3 cups grated cheddar cheese

Salt and black pepper to taste

Directions and Total Time: approx. 20 minutes

Melt butter in a pot and saute onion and garlic for 3 minutes. Add salt and pepper to taste. Add broccoli, broth and bring to a boil. Reduce the heat, and simmer until the soup is ready to serve for 10 mins. Blend the soup with an immersion blender until it is smooth. Add 2 cups of cheese and cook for one minute. Mix in heavy cream. Serve topped with cheddar cheese.

Per serving: Cal 561; Net Carbs 7g; Fat 52g; Protein 24g

Slow Cooked Sausage Soup with Beer

Ingredients for 8 servings

1 cup heavy cream

10 oz beef sausages, sliced

1 cup chopped celery

1 cup chopped carrots

4 garlic cloves, minced

8 ounces cream cheese

1 tsp red pepper flakes

6 ounces beer

16 ounces beef stock

1 onion, diced

1 cups cheddar cheese

3 tbsp chopped cilantro

Directions and Total Time: approx. 8 hours

Add the broth, beer and sausage, as well as carrots, celery, onion red pepper, flakes and pepper, salt to a slow cooker, and mix to zcombine. Add enough water to cover the ingredients with 2 inches. Cover the pot to cook 6 hours at a low temperature. Stir in heavy cream, cheddar, and cream cheeses and cook for 2 hours. Ladle the soup into bowls and garnish with cilantro.

Per serving: Cal 244; Net Carbs 4g; Fat 17g, Protein 5g

Red Gazpacho

Ingredients for 6 servings

2 green peppers, roasted

2 large red peppers, roasted

2 avocados, flesh scoped out

2 garlic cloves

2 spring onions, chopped

1 cucumber, chopped

1 cup olive oil

2 tbsp lemon juice

4 tomatoes, chopped

7 ounces goat cheese

1 red onion, coarsely chopped

2 tbsp apple cider vinegar

Directions and Total Time: approx. 10 min + chilling time

Place the tomatoes, peppers, spring onions, avocado, garlic, lemon juice, vinegar, oil, and salt in the food processor. Then, pulse until it becomes slightly chunky but still smooth. Adjust the seasoning, then transfer the mixture to a pot. Mix in the red onion and cucumbers. Cover and refrigerate for at least 2 hours. Serve chilled, topped by goat cheese, and sprinkle of olive oil.

Per serving: Cal 528; Net Carbs 8.5g; Fat 46g,

Protein 7g

Superfood & Low-Protein Soup

Ingredients for 6 servings

1 broccoli head, chopped

7 ounces spinach

1 onion, chopped

2 garlic cloves, minced

5 ounces watercress

4 cups veggie stock

1 cup coconut milk

1 tbsp ghee

1 bay leaf

Salt and black pepper to taste

Directions and Total Time: approx. 20 minutes

Melt ghee in a saucepan at medium-high temperature. Add garlic and onion, then cook them for three minutes. Add broccoli, stir and cook for another 5 minutes. Mix the broth and the bay leaf. Then, bring to the boil. Reduce the heat, and cook until 3 mins. Add watercress and spinach then cook 3 mins. Stir in coconut cream and salt and pepper. Remove the bay leaf then blend it using the aid of a hand blender. Serve the soup cold.

Per serving: Cal 392; Net Carbs 5.8g; Fat 38g, Protein 5g

Chicken Enchilada Soup

Ingredients for 4 servings

½ cup salsa enchilada verde

2 cups cooked shredded chicken

2 cups chicken broth

1 cup grated cheddar cheese

4 ounces cream cheese

½ tsp chili powder

½ tsp ground cumin

½ tsp fresh cilantro, chopped

Directions and Total Time: approx. 15 minutes

Mix salsa verde and cream cheese along with broth into a processor. process until the mixture is smooth. Transfer the mixture to a pot. Heat until the water is the water is hot, but do not bring to a boil. Add the chicken along with chili powder, cumin and cook for 5 minutes. Mix in cheddar cheese and season according to your preference. Serve with cilantro sprinkled on top.

Per serving: Cal 346; Net Carbs 3g; Fat 23g, Protein 25g

Creamy Chicken Soup

Ingredients for 4 servings

2 cups shredded cooked chicken

3 tbsp butter, melted

4 cups chicken broth

4 tbsp chopped cilantro

⅓ cup buffalo sauce

4 ounces cream cheese

Directions and Total Time: approx. 15 minutes

Blend the buffalo sauce, butter and cream cheese in a food processor until it is uniform and smooth. Transfer to a saucepan. Place the chicken in the pot, add the broth, and simmer until the chicken is cooked. Serve with garnishes of cilantro.

Per serving: Cal 406; Net Carbs 5g; Fat 29.5g, Protein 26g

Coconut Cream Pumpkin Soup

Ingredients for 4 servings

2 red onions, cut into wedges

2 garlic cloves

10 oz pumpkin, cubed

10 oz butternut squash, cubed

2 tbsp melted vegan butter

8 oz vegan butter

Salt and black pepper to taste

Juice of 1 lime

¾ cup vegan mayonnaise

Toasted pumpkin seeds

Directions and Total Time: approx. 55 minutes

Pre-heat oven to 400 F. Add onions as well as pumpkin and squash on an oven-proof baking sheet. Drizzle with butter that has melted. Sprinkle with salt and pepper. Cook for 30 to 45 minutes, or until the vegetables are delicious and golden brown. Transfer them to a saucepan. Add 2 cups of water and bring to a boil, then simmer up to 15 mins. Break the remaining vegan butter in the pot. Puree the vegetables until it is smooth. Add lime juice and vegan mayonnaise. Serve with pumpkin seeds.

Per serving: Cal 643; Fat 57g; Net Carbs 9g; Protein 10g

Reuben Soup

Ingredients for 6 servings

1 onion, diced

7 cups beef stock

1 tsp caraway seeds

2 celery stalks, diced

2 garlic cloves, minced

¾ tsp black pepper

2 cups heavy cream

1 cup sauerkraut

1 pound corned beef, chopped

3 tbsp butter

1 ½ cups Swiss cheese

Salt and black pepper to taste

Directions and Total Time: approx. 30 minutes

Melt butter in a large pot. Add celery and onions and cook for 3 minutes until they are tender. Add garlic and cook for a further minute. Then pour the soup over, and mix in sauerkraut, salt, and caraway seeds, and the pinch of pepper. Bring to a boil. Lower the temperature to a simmer, and then add the corned beef. Cook for around 15 minutes. Make adjustments to the spice. Mix in the heavy cream and Swiss cheese, and cook for one minute. Serve.

Per serving: Cal 450; Net Carbs 8g; Fat 37g, Protein 23g

Chorizo & Cauliflower Soup

Ingredients for 4 servings

1 cauliflower head, chopped

1 turnip, chopped

3 tbsp butter

1 chorizo sausage, sliced

2 cups chicken broth

1 small onion, chopped

2 cups water

Salt and black pepper to taste

Directions and Total Time: approx. 40 minutes

Melt 2 tbsp of butter in a pot. Add onions, stirring until tender and golden about 6 minutes. Add the turnip and cauliflower and cook for 5 minutes. Add broth. Bring to a boil, simmer, and cook for 20 minutes. Melt the remaining butter in a skillet. Then add the chorizo in 5 minutes and let it cook. Blend the soup with the aid of a hand blender until it is smooth. Adjust the seasonings. Serve in large bowls, topped with the chorizo.

Per serving: Cal 251; Net Carbs 5.7g; Fat 19g, Protein 10g

Ginger-Spinach Egg Benedict Soup

Ingredients for 4 servings

2 tbsp butter

1 tbsp sesame oil

1 small onion, finely sliced

3 garlic cloves, minced

2 tsp ginger paste

2 cups baby spinach, chopped

2 cups chopped green beans

4 cups vegetable stock

3 tbsp chopped cilantro

4 eggs

Directions and Total Time: approx. 35 minutes

Melt butter in a pot and saute onions, garlic, and ginger for 4 minutes, stirring frequently. Mix spinach, allowing to wilt. Pour in the green beans and stock. Bring the soup to a boil, then reduce the heat, then allow to simmer for 10 mins. Transfer the soup into the blender and blend until smooth. Bring 3 cups of vinegared water to a simmer. When it's warm, pour in an egg and allow it to cook for 3 minutes remove with a perforated spoon. Repeat this process with the remaining eggs, one at each. Divide the soup among four bowls, and then place

eggs on each bowl and drizzle it with sesame oil and garnish with cilantro and serve.

Per serving: Cal 463; Net Carbs 5.8g; Fat 30g, Protein 23g

Spinach & Poached Egg Soup

Ingredients for 4 servings

1 tbsp olive oil

2 tbsp butter

1 red onion, thinly sliced

3 garlic cloves, finely sliced

4 cups spinach, chopped

1 lettuce head, chopped

4 cups vegetable stock

6 sprigs parsley

1 tbsp fresh dill for garnishing

Salt and black pepper to taste

4 eggs

1 cup grated Parmesan cheese

Directions and Total Time: approx. 35 minutes

Heat butter and oil in a pot and saute onions and garlic for three minutes. Mix in the lettuce and spinach to cook 5 mins. Add vegetable stock; bring to a boil. Reduce the heat and allow the soup to simmer for at least 10 minutes. By using an immersion blender blend the soup until it is smooth. Add salt and pepper to taste. Make 1 cup of the water simmer in a different saucepan. Create a whirlpool at the middle using an wooden spoon. Let the water return to normal, and then crack an egg. Poach for three minutes, then take it out and place on an oven-safe dish. Repeat poaching the eggs for 3 minutes, then remove and set aside. Divide the soup between serving bowls. Top with poached eggs. Decorate with dill and Parmesan cheese and serve hot.

Per serving: Cal 515; Net Carbs 4.5g; Fat 33g, Protein 38g

Rosemary Onion Soup

Ingredients for 4 servings

2 tbsp butter

1 tbsp olive oil

3 cups sliced white onions

2 garlic cloves, thinly sliced

2 tsp almond flour

½ cup dry white wine

2 sprigs chopped rosemary

Salt and black pepper to taste

2 cups almond milk

1 cup grated Parmesan cheese

Directions and Total Time: approx. 35 minutes

Heat butter and oil in a pot and saute onions and garlic for 6-7 minutes. Turn the flame down to a simmer and cook for another 10 minutes. Mix in the flour, wine, salt, pepper, rosemary, salt and add 2 cups of water. Bring to a boil, then allow to simmer 10 minutes. Pour in the milk aswell as half the Parmesan cheese. Stir to melt the cheese and spoon into a serving bowl. Top with the remaining Parmesan cheese and serve.

Per serving: Cal 340; Net Carbs 5.6g; Fat 23g, Protein 15g

Wild Mushroom Soup

Ingredients for 4 servings

12 oz wild mushrooms, chopped

¼ cup butter

5 ounces crème fraiche

2 tsp thyme leaves

2 garlic cloves, minced

4 cups chicken broth

Salt and black pepper to taste

Directions and Total Time: approx. 30 minutes

Melt butter in a large pot over medium heat. Add garlic and cook for one minute until it is it is tender. Add the mushrooms, season with salt and pepper then cook until cooked for nine minutes. Pour the broth over and bring to a boil. Reduce the heat and let it simmer until it is 10 mins. Blend using a hand mixer until the mixture is smooth. Stir in creme Fraiche. Serve garnished with thyme.

Per serving: Cal 281; Net Carbs 5.8g; Fat 25g, Protein 6g

Spinach & Kale Soup with Fried Collards

Ingredients for 4 servings

3 oz vegan butter

1 cup spinach, coarsely

1 cup kale, coarsely

1 large avocado

3 ½ cups coconut cream

1 cup vegetable broth

3 tbsp chopped mint leaves

Juice from 1 lime

1 cup collard greens, chopped

3 garlic cloves, minced

3 tbsp green cardamom powder

Toasted pistachios

Directions and Total Time: approx. 15 minutes

Set a saucepan and melt vegan butter. Add kale and spinach and cook in 5 mins. Transfer to the food processor. Add avocado, coconut cream, mint, lime juice, salt and pepper. Puree until smooth. Reserve the soup. Heat the saucepan again with butter and add collards greens, garlic, as well as cardamom. Cook for four minutes. Pour into bowls and decorate with a few scoops of collards and pistachios.

Per serving: Cal 885; Fat 80g; Net Carbs 15g; Protein 14g

Tofu Goulash Soup

Ingredients for 4 servings

1 ½ cups tofu, crumbled

4 ¼ oz vegan butter

1 white onion

2 garlic cloves

8 oz chopped butternut squash

1 red bell pepper

1 tbsp paprika powder

¼ tsp red chili flakes

1 tbsp dried basil

Salt and black pepper to taste

1 ½ cups crushed tomatoes

3 cups vegetable broth

1 ½ tsp red wine vinegar

Chopped cilantro to serve

Directions and Total Time: approx. 25 minutes

Melt vegan butter in a pot set over medium heat and saute onion and garlic for 3 minutes until fragrant and soft. Add tofu to the mix then cook it for three minutes. Add bell pepper, squash red chili flakes, paprika and basil, salt and pepper. Cook until tender for two minutes. Add the tomatoes and broth. Cover the lid and bring to a boil, then reduce the heat to simmer for 10 minutes; mix in vinegar. Garnish with cilantro and serve.

Per serving: Cal 481; Fat 41.8g; Net Carbs 9g; Protein 12g

Celery Dill Soup

Ingredients for 4 servings

1 small head cauliflower, cut into florets

2 tbsp coconut oil

½ lb celery root, chopped

1 garlic clove

1 white onion, sliced

¼ cup dill, roughly chopped

1 tsp cumin powder

¼ tsp nutmeg powder

3 ½ cups vegetable stock

5 oz butter

Juice from 1 lemon

¼ cup coconut cream

Salt and black pepper to taste

Directions and Total Time: approx. 25 minutes

Heat coconut oil in a saucepan over medium heat. Once the coconut oil has warmed, add celery root, garlic clove and onion to the pan and cook for 5 minutes. Add the cumin, dill, and nutmeg, and fry for another minute. Add the cauliflorets and stock. Let the soup boil for 15 minutes. Turn off the heat. Add butter and lemon juice. Blend the ingredients in an immersion blender until smooth. Mix in coconut cream and season to taste. Spoon into bowls and serve warm.

Per serving: Cal 410; Fat 37g; Net Carbs 9g; Protein

6g

Broccoli Fennel Soup

Ingredients for 4 servings

1 fennel bulb, chopped

10 oz broccoli, cut into florets

3 cups vegetable stock

Salt and black pepper to taste

1 garlic clove

1 cup cream cheese

3 oz butter

½ cup chopped fresh oregano

Directions and Total Time: approx. 25 minutes

Put fennel, broccoli, and garlic in a pot and cover with stock. Bring to a boil on medium heat. Cook for 17 minutes. Season the mixture with salt and pepper. Pour in cream cheese, butter, and oregano; puree the ingredients with an immersion blender until smooth. Serve with vegan cheese crackers.

Per serving: Cal 510; Fat 44g; Net Carbs 7g; Protein 16g

Parsnip-Tomato Soup

Ingredients for 4 servings

1 tbsp butter

1 tbsp olive oil

1 large red onion, chopped

4 garlic cloves, minced

6 red bell peppers, sliced

1 daikon radish, chopped

2 parsnips, chopped

3 cups chopped tomatoes

4 cups vegetable stock

3 cups coconut milk

2 cups toasted chopped walnuts

1 cup grated Parmesan cheese

Directions and Total Time: approx. 40 minutes

In a large saucepan, heat butter and olive oil. Sauté onion and garlic for three minutes. Cook for 10 minutes. Stir in bell peppers and daikon radish. Add tomatoes and stock. Let simmer for 20 minutes. Blend the soup using an immersion blender. Stir in the coconut milk. Serve with Parmesan cheese and walnuts.

Per serving: Cal 955; Net Carbs 4g; Fat 86g, Protein 19.1g

Mixed Mushroom Soup

Ingredients for 4 servings

5 oz white button mushrooms, chopped

5 oz cremini mushrooms, chopped

5 oz shiitake mushrooms, chopped

4 oz unsalted butter

1 small onion, finely chopped

1 clove garlic, minced

½ lb celery root, chopped

½ tsp dried rosemary

4 cups water

1 vegan stock cube, crushed

1 tbsp plain vinegar

1 cup coconut cream

6 leaves basil, chopped

Directions and Total Time: approx. 35 minutes

In a saucepan, melt butter. Sauté onion, garlic and mushrooms in butter until fragrant and golden brown, approximately 6 minutes. Reserve some mushrooms for garnishing. Mix in the vinegar, water, stock cube and rosemary. Bring to a boil and stir for 6 minutes. Reduce heat to low and simmer for 15 mins. Add coconut cream to the mixture and blend. Spoon into bowls garnished with the reserved mushrooms and basil.

Per serving: Cal 506; Fat 46g; Net Carbs 12g; Protein 8g

Creamy Tofu Soup

Ingredients for 4 servings

1 cup cremini mushrooms, sliced and pre-cooked

1 tbsp olive oil

1 garlic clove, minced

1 white onion, finely chopped

1 tsp ginger puree

1 cup vegetable stock

2 turnips, peeled and chopped

Salt and black pepper to taste

2 (14 oz) silken tofu, drained

2 cups almond milk

1 tbsp chopped basil

Finely chopped parsley

Chopped walnuts for topping

Directions and Total Time: approx. 25 minutes

In a large saucepan, heat olive oil and fry garlic, onion, ginger, until softened, approximately 3 minutes. Add in the stock and turnip. Season with salt and pepper. Cook for 6 minutes. Blend the ingredients with an immersion blender until smooth. Add in the mushrooms, and cook covered for 7 minutes. Heat milk for 2 minutes. Add basil and parsley to the mixture and stir.

Per serving: Cal 923; Net Carbs 7.4g; Fat 8.5g, Protein 23g

Spring Vegetable Soup

Ingredients for 4 servings

4 cups vegetable stock

1 cup pearl onions, halved

3 cups green beans, chopped

2 cups asparagus, chopped

2 cups baby spinach

1 tbsp garlic powder

Salt and white pepper to taste

2 cups grated Parmesan

Directions and Total Time: approx. 25 minutes

In a large pot, heat vegetable broth. Add pearl onions, green beans and asparagus. Cook for 10 minutes. Season the soup with salt, white pepper, and garlic powder. Allow spinach to wilt slightly before adding in. Serve with Parmesan cheese.

Per serving: Cal 196; Net Carbs 4.3g; Fat 12g, Protein 2.5g

Chilled Lemongrass & Avocado Soup

Ingredients for 4 servings

4 cups chopped avocado pulp

2 stalks lemongrass, chopped

4 cups vegetable broth

2 lemons, juiced

3 tbsp chopped mint

2 cups heavy cream

Directions and Total Time: approx. 20 min + chilling time

Let the broth, avocado, and lemongrass boil in a saucepan over low heat for 10 min. Add in the lemon juice and heat off. Blend the ingredients with an immersion blender. Add in the heavy cream. Pour into bowls. Chill for one hour. Serve with mint leaves

Per serving: Cal 339; Net Carbs 3.5g; Fat 33g, Protein 3.5g

Herby Cheese & Bacon Soup

Ingredients for 4 servings

1 tbsp olive oil

6 slices bacon, chopped

4 tbsp butter

1 small white onion, chopped

3 garlic cloves, minced

2 tbsp finely chopped thyme

1 tbsp chopped fresh tarragon

1 tbsp chopped fresh oregano

2 cups cubed parsnips

3 ½ cups vegetable broth

Salt and black pepper to taste

1 cup almond milk

1 cup grated cheddar cheese

2 tbsp chopped scallions

Directions and Total Time: approx. 25 minutes

In a saucepan, heat olive oil and fry bacon for 5 minutes. In a saucepan, melt butter. Once the butter has melted, saute onion and garlic for 3 minutes. Season the parsnips with salt and pepper and let them cook for 12 minutes, until they soften. Blend the soup with an immersion blender until smooth. Add milk and cheese to the soup and continue stirring constantly until it melts. Serve with bacon and scallions.

Per serving: Cal 775; Net Carbs 6.5g; Fat 57g, Protein 18g

Pork & Pumpkin Stew

Ingredients for 6 servings

1 cup pumpkin puree

2 lb chopped pork stew meat

1 tbsp peanut butter

4 tbsp chopped peanuts

1 garlic clove, minced

½ cup chopped onion

½ cup white wine

1 tbsp olive oil

1 tsp lemon juice

¼ cup granulated sweetener

¼ tsp cardamom powder

¼ tsp allspice

2 cups water

2 cups chicken stock

Directions and Total Time: approx. 45 minutes

In a saucepan, heat olive oil and saute garlic and onion for 3 minutes. Cook the pork for 5-6 minutes. Add the wine to the pot and let it simmer for about 1 minute. Mix in all the other ingredients except for lemon juice and peanuts. Bring to boil. Cook for 5 minutes. Reduce heat to low, and simmer for 30 minutes. Adjust the seasonings and add the lemon. Top with peanuts.

Per serving: Cal 451, Net Carbs: 4g, Fat: 33g, Protein: 27g

Asparagus & Shrimp Curry Soup

Ingredients for 4 servings

2 tbsp ghee

1 lb jumbo shrimp, deveined

2 tsp ginger-garlic puree

2 tbsp red curry paste

6 oz coconut milk

1 bunch asparagus

Directions and Total Time: approx. 20 minutes

In a saucepan, melt the ghee and add shrimp. Season the shrimp with salt and chili pepper, and cook for three minutes. Transfer to a plate. Stir in the ginger-garlic paste and red curry paste and cook for 2 minutes. Add coconut milk, asparagus and shrimp to the ghee. Cook for 4 minutes. Reduce heat to low and simmer for three minutes more. Serve with cauli rice.

Per serving: Cal 375; Net Carbs 2g; Fat 35.4g, Protein 9g

Thyme Tomato Soup

Ingredients for 6 servings

2 tbsp butter

2 large red onions, diced

½ cup raw cashew nuts, diced

2 (28-oz) cans tomatoes

1 tsp thyme

1 ½ cups water

Salt and black pepper to taste

1 cup half-and-half

Directions and Total Time: approx. 20 minutes

In a large saucepan, melt butter and cook the onion for four minutes. Add tomatoes, thyme and water. Season with salt and pepper. Simmer for 10 minutes. Blend the ingredients using an immersion blender. Mix in the half-and-half to adjust the flavor. Serve in soup bowls.

Per serving: Cal 310; Net Carbs 3g; Fat 27g, Protein 11g

Cauliflower Soup with Kielbasa

Ingredients for 4 servings

1 cauliflower head, chopped

1 rutabaga, chopped

3 tbsp ghee

1 kielbasa sausage, sliced

2 cups chicken broth

1 small onion, chopped

2 cups water

Salt and black pepper, to taste

Directions and Total Time: approx. 40 minutes

In a saucepan, heat 2 tablespoons of the ghee and sauté the onion for 3 minutes. Cook for 5 more minutes. Add the cauliflower and rutabaga. Add broth, water, and salt. Add salt and pepper to taste. Bring to boil. Cook for 20 minutes. In a large skillet, melt the butter. Cook the kielbasa sausage for 5 minutes. Blend the soup until smooth. Serve the soup with kielbasa.

Per serving: Cal 251; Net Carbs: 5.7g; Fat: 19g, Protein: 10g

Tomato Soup with Parmesan Croutons

Ingredients for 6 servings

Parmesan Croutons:

3 tbsp flax seed powder

1¼ cups almond flour

2 tsp baking powder

5 tbsp psyllium husk powder

1¼ cups boiling water

2 tsp plain vinegar

3 oz butter

2 oz grated Parmesan

Tomato Soup

2 lb fresh ripe tomatoes

4 cloves garlic, peeled only

1 small white onion, diced

1 red bell pepper, diced

3 tbsp olive oil

1 cup coconut cream

½ tsp dried rosemary

½ tsp dried oregano

2 tbsp chopped fresh basil

Salt and black pepper to taste

Directions and Total Time: approx. 1 hour 25 minutes

For the parmesan croutons:

In a bowl, mix the flax seed powder with 2/3 cup of water and set aside for 5 minutes. Pre-heat oven to

350 F. Line a baking sheet with parchment. Combine almond flour, baking powder and psyllium powder in a separate bowl. Combine the boiling water with the plain vinegar. Mix in the flour mixture. Continue to whisk for 30 seconds, until it is well combined. Make 8 flat pieces from the dough. Place the dough on a baking sheet, leaving enough space between each piece to allow for rising. Bake for 40 minutes. Allow croutons cool to room temperature before slicing into halves. Spread butter and Parmesan mixture inside the croutons. Bake for five minutes.

For the tomato soup:

Add tomatoes, onion, bell pepper and garlic to a large pan. Drizzle olive oil over the top. After 25 minutes of roasting, broil the vegetables for 4 minutes. Blend until smooth. Add coconut cream, rosemary and oregano, salt, pepper to the blender. Blend until smooth. Serve with croutons.

Per serving: Cal 434; Fat 38g; Net Carbs 6g; Protein 11g

Colby Cauliflower Soup with Pancetta Chips

Ingredients for 4 servings

2 heads cauliflower, cut into florets

2 tbsp ghee

1 onion, chopped

2 cups water

3 cups almond milk

1 cup Colby cheese, shredded

3 pancetta strips

Directions and Total Time: approx. 30 minutes

In a saucepan, melt the ghee and cook the onion for 3 minutes. Add cauliflorets and saute for 3 more minutes. Season with salt and pepper. Bring to a boil. Reduce heat and simmer for 10 minutes. Blend cauliflower until smooth. Add almond milk and cheese to melt the cheese. Taste. In a skillet, fry pancetta until crispy. Serve the soup with pancetta crispy.

Per serving: Cal 402; Net Carbs 6g; Fat 37g; Protein 8g

Coconut Turkey Chili

Ingredients for 4 servings

1 pound turkey breasts, cubed

1 cup broccoli, chopped

2 shallots, sliced

1 (14-ounce) can tomatoes

2 tbsp coconut oil

2 tbsp coconut cream

2 garlic cloves, minced

1 tbsp ground coriander

2 tbsp fresh ginger, grated

1 tbsp turmeric

1 tbsp cumin

2 tbsp chili powder

Directions and Total Time: approx. 30 minutes

Heat coconut oil in a saucepan over medium heat. Stir-fry turkeys, shallots and garlic for five minutes. Stir in tomatoes, broccoli, turmeric, coriander, cumin, chili, salt and pepper. Cook for 20-25 minutes. Blend in a food processor. Serve.

Per serving: Cal 318; Net Carbs 6.6g; Fat 18.7g; Protein 27g

Effortless Chicken Chili

Ingredients for 4 servings

1 tbsp butter

1 tbsp sesame oil

¼ tsp ginger, ground

4 chicken tenders, cubed

1 onion, chopped

2 cups chicken broth

8 oz diced tomatoes

2 oz tomato paste

1 tbsp cumin

1 red chili pepper, minced

½ cup shredded cheddar

Salt and black pepper to taste

Directions and Total Time: approx. 30 minutes

Put a pan and add chicken. Bring to a boil. Cook for 10 minutes. Transfer the cooked vegetables to a plate and mash them with forks. Put butter and sesame oil in a saucepan and cook onion and ginger for five minutes. Stir in chicken, tomatoes, cumin, red chili pepper, tomato paste, and broth. Bring the mixture to boil. Reduce heat to low and simmer for 10 minutes. Serve with cheddar cheese.

Per serving: Cal 396; Net Carbs 5.7g; Fat 22.9g; Protein 38g

Cauliflower Beef Curry

Ingredients for 4 servings

1 head cauliflower, cut into florets

2 tbsp olive oil

1 ½ pounds ground beef

1 tbsp ginger-garlic paste

½ tsp cumin

¼ tsp allspice

6 oz canned whole tomatoes

Salt and chili pepper to taste

Directions and Total Time: approx. 26 minutes

Cook beef in hot oil over medium heat for 5 minutes while breaking any lumps. Add cumin, allspice and salt. Cover the pan with tomatoes and cauliflower and let it cook for 6 minutes. Bring to a boil 1/4 cup water. Cook on medium heat for 10 minutes, or until water is half-boiled. Adjust the taste with salt. Serve warm.

Per serving: Cal 518; Net Carbs 3g; Fat 34.6g; Protein 44.6g

Chicken Stew with Spinach

Ingredients for 4 servings

28 oz chicken thighs, skinless, boneless

2 oz sun-dried tomatoes, chopped

2 carrots, chopped

2 tbsp olive oil

2 celery stalks, chopped

2 cups chicken stock

1 leek, chopped

3 garlic cloves, minced

½ tsp dried rosemary

1 cup spinach

¼ tsp dried thyme

½ cup heavy cream

Salt and black pepper to taste

A pinch of xanthan gum

Directions and Total Time: approx. 50 minutes

Heat olive oil in a large pot. Add garlic, carrots and celery to the pot. Season with salt and pepper. Sauté for 5-6 minutes. Cook the chicken for 5 minutes. Add in the stock, tomatoes and rosemary, thyme and simmer for 30 minutes. Cook for 5 minutes. Add the cream, xanthan gum and spinach. Serve.

Per serving: Cal 224, Net Carbs 6g, Fat 11g, Protein 23g

Bacon Stew with Cauliflower

Ingredients for 6 servings

1 head cauliflower, cut into florets

8 oz grated mozzarella

2 cups chicken broth

½ tsp garlic powder

½ tsp onion powder

Salt and black pepper, to taste

4 garlic cloves, minced

¼ cup heavy cream

3 cups bacon, chopped

Directions and Total Time: approx. 40 minutes

In a pot, combine the bacon with broth, cauliflower, salt, heavy cream, black pepper, garlic powder, cheese, onion powder, and garlic, and cook for 35 minutes. Serve.

Per serving: Cal 380; Net Carbs 6g; Fat 25g; Protein 33g

Scottish Beef Stew

Ingredients for 4 servings

12 oz sweet potatoes, cut into quarters

2 tbsp lard

1 ¼ lb beef chuck roast, cubed

1 parsnip, chopped

1 onion, chopped

1 clove garlic, minced

Salt and black pepper to taste

1 ½ cups beef stock

2 tsp rosemary, chopped

Directions and Total Time: approx. 60 minutes

Heat lard in skillet on medium heat. Add onion and garlic to skillet and cook for 4 minutes. Season the beef with salt and pepper and cook for 7-8 minutes. Add the sweet potatoes, parsnips, rosemary, and beef broth. Cover and stir. Cook on low heat for 35-40 mins. Serve.

Per serving: Cal 445; Net Carbs 12.3g; Fat 18g; Protein 42g

Vegetable Stew

Ingredients for 4 servings

1 large head broccoli, cut into florets

2 tbsp ghee

1 tbsp onion-garlic puree

4 medium carrots, chopped

2 cups green beans, halved

1 cup water

1 ½ cups heavy cream

Directions and Total Time: approx. 35 minutes

Melt ghee in a saucepan and sauté onion-garlic puree for 2 minutes. Stir in carrots, broccoli, and green beans, salt, and pepper, add water, stir again, and cook for 25 minutes. Mix in heavy cream, turn the heat off and adjust the taste. Serve the stew with almond flour bread.

Per serving: Cal 310; Net Carbs 6g; Fat 26.4g; Protein 8g

Chili Beef Stew with Cauliflower Grits

Ingredients for 4 servings

2 tbsp olive oil

2 lb chuck roast, cubed

1 large yellow onion, chopped

3 garlic cloves, minced

2 large tomatoes, diced

1 tbsp rosemary

1 tbsp smoked paprika

2 tsp chili powder

2 cups beef broth

2 tbsp butter

½ cup walnuts, chopped

2 cups cauliflower rice

1 cup half and half

1 cup shredded cheddar

Directions and Total Time: approx. 55 minutes

Heat olive oil in a pot. Season beef with salt and pepper and cook for 3 minutes. Stir in onion, garlic, and tomatoes, for 5 minutes. Mix in rosemary, paprika, chili and cook for 2 minutes. Pour in broth and bring to a boil, then simmer for 25 minutes; set aside. Melt butter in a pot, and cook walnuts for 3 minutes. Transfer to a cutting board, chop and plate. Pour cauli rice and ½ cup water into the pot and cook for 5 minutes. Stir in half and half for 3 minutes. Mix in cheddar cheese, fold in walnuts. Top with stewed beef.

Per serving: Cal 736; Net Carbs 7.8g; Fat 48g, Protein 63g

Rustic Lamb Stew with Root Veggies

Ingredients for 4 servings

2 tbsp olive oil

1 pound lamb chops

1 garlic clove, minced

1 parsnip, chopped

1 onion, chopped

1 celery stalk, chopped

Salt and black pepper to taste

2 cups vegetable stock

2 carrots, chopped

½ tbsp rosemary, chopped

1 tbsp sweet paprika

1 leek, chopped

1 tbsp tomato paste

½ fennel bulb, chopped

Directions and Total Time: approx. 1 hour 45

minutes

Warm olive oil in a pot over medium heat and cook celery, onion, leek, and garlic for 5 minutes. Add in lamb chops, and cook for 4 minutes. Add in paprika, carrots, parsnip, fennel, stock, tomato paste; let simmer for 1 hour. Adjust the seasoning, sprinkle with rosemary, and serve.

Per serving: Cal 472; Net Carbs 6.3g; Fat 37g; Protein 20.5g

Beef & Veggie Stew

Ingredients for 4 servings

1 pound ground beef

2 tbsp olive oil

1 onion, chopped

2 garlic cloves, minced

14 oz canned diced tomatoes

1 tbsp dried sage

Salt and black pepper, to taste

2 carrots, sliced

2 celery stalks, chopped

1 cup vegetable broth

Directions and Total Time: approx. 30 minutes

Warm olive oil in a pan and sauté onion, celery, and garlic for 5 minutes. Add in beef and cook for 6 minutes. Pour in tomatoes, carrots, broth, pepper, salt, and sage, lower the heat and simmer for 15 minutes.

Per serving: Cal 253, Net Carbs 5.2g, Fat 13g, Protein 30g

Veal Stew

Ingredients for 6 servings

3 lb veal shoulder, cubed

2 tbsp olive oil

1 onion, chopped

1 garlic clove, minced

1 ½ cups red wine

12 oz canned tomato sauce

1 carrot, chopped

1 cup mushrooms, chopped

½ cup green beans

2 tsp dried oregano

Directions and Total Time: approx. 120 minutes

Warm olive oil in a pot and brown the veal for 5-6 minutes. Stir in onion and garlic and cook for 3 minutes. Place in wine, oregano, carrot, pepper, salt, tomato sauce, 1 cup water, and mushrooms and bring to a boil. Reduce the heat to low and cook for 1 hour and 45 minutes, then add in green beans and cook for 5 minutes. Serve.

Per serving: Cal 415, Net Carbs 5.2g, Fat 21g, Protein 44g

Turkey Stew with Tomatillo Salsa

Ingredients for 6 servings

4 cups leftover turkey meat, chopped

2 cups green beans

6 cups chicken stock

Salt and black pepper to taste

1 chipotle pepper, chopped

½ cup tomatillo salsa

1 tsp ground coriander

2 tsp cumin

¼ cup sour cream

1 tbsp fresh cilantro, chopped

Directions and Total Time: approx. 30 minutes

Set a pan over medium heat. Add in the stock and heat. Stir in green beans, and cook for 10 minutes. Place in turkey, ground coriander, salt, tomatillo salsa, chipotle pepper, cumin, and black pepper, and cook for 10 minutes. Stir in the sour cream, kill the heat, and separate into bowls. Top with chopped cilantro to serve.

Per serving: Cal 193, Net Carbs 2g, Fat 11g, Protein 27g

Pork & Pumpkin Stew with Peanuts

Ingredients for 6 servings

1 cup puree

2 lb pork shoulder, cubed

1 tbsp peanut butter

4 tbsp chopped peanuts

1 garlic clove, minced

½ cup chopped onion

½ cup white wine

1 tbsp olive oil

1 tsp lemon juice

¼ cup granulated sweetener

¼ tsp cardamom

¼ tsp allspice

3 cups chicken stock

Salt and black pepper to taste

Directions and Total Time: approx. 45 minutes

Heat olive oil in a pot. Add onions and garlic and sauté for 3 minutes. Add in pork and stir-fry for 5-6 minutes. Pour in wine and cook for 1 minute. Throw in the remaining ingredients, except lemon juice and peanuts. Bring the mixture to a boil, and cook for 5 minutes. Reduce the heat and let cook for 30 minutes. Adjust seasoning. Stir in lemon juice before serving. Serve topped with peanuts.

Per serving: Cal 451; Net Carbs 4g; Fat 33g, Protein 27.5g

Paprika Chicken & Bacon Stew

Ingredients for 3 servings

8 bacon strips, chopped

¼ cup Dijon mustard

Salt and black pepper to taste

1 onion, chopped

1 tbsp olive oil

1 ½ cups chicken stock

3 chicken breasts

¼ tsp sweet paprika

Directions and Total Time: approx. 40 minutes

In a bowl, combine salt, pepper, and mustard. Massage onto chicken breasts. Set a pan over medium heat, stir in the bacon, cook until it browns, and remove to a plate. Heat oil in the same pan, add the breasts, cook each side for 2 minutes, set aside. Place in the stock and bring to a simmer. Stir in pancetta and onions. Return the chicken to the pan as well, stir gently, and simmer for 20 minutes over medium heat, turning halfway

through. Serve.

Per serving: Cal 313; Net Carbs 3g; Fat 18g, Protein 26g

Parsley Sausage Stew

Ingredients for 6 servings

1 lb pork sausage, sliced

1 red bell pepper, chopped

1 onion, chopped

Salt and black pepper, to taste

1 cup fresh parsley, chopped

6 green onions, chopped

¼ cup avocado oil

1 cup chicken stock

2 garlic cloves, minced

24 ounces canned tomatoes

16 ounces okra, sliced

6 ounces tomato sauce

2 tbsp coconut aminos

1 tbsp hot sauce

Directions and Total Time: approx. 35 minutes

Set a pot over medium heat and warm oil. Place in sausages and cook for 2 minutes. Stir in onion, green onions, garlic, black pepper, bell pepper, and salt, and cook for 5 minutes. Add in hot sauce, stock, tomatoes, coconut aminos, okra, and tomato sauce, bring to a simmer and cook for 15 minutes. Sprinkle with fresh parsley to serve.

Per serving: Cal 314, Net Carbs 7g, Fat 25g, Protein 16g

Brazilian Moqueca (Shrimp Stew)

Ingredients for 6 servings

1 ½ pounds shrimp, peeled and deveined

1 cup coconut milk

2 tbsp lime juice

¼ cup diced roasted peppers

3 tbsp olive oil

1 garlic clove, minced

14 ounces diced tomatoes

2 tbsp harissa sauce

1 chopped onion

¼ cup chopped cilantro

Salt and black pepper to taste

Directions and Total Time: approx. 25 minutes

Warm olive oil in a pot and sauté onion and garlic for 3 minutes. Add in tomatoes and shrimp. Cook for 3-4 minutes. Stir in harissa sauce, roasted peppers, and coconut milk and cook for 2 minutes. Add in lime juice and season with salt and pepper. Top with cilantro to serve.

Per serving: Cal 324; Net Carbs 5g; Fats 21g; Protein 23g

Yellow Squash Duck Breast Stew

Ingredients for 2 servings

1 pound duck breast, skin on and sliced

2 yellow squash, sliced

1 tbsp coconut oil

1 green onion bunch, chopped

1 carrot, chopped

2 green bell peppers, chopped

Salt and black pepper, to taste

Directions and Total Time: approx. 20 minutes

Set a pan over high heat and warm oil, stir in the green onions, and cook for 2 minutes. Place in the yellow squash, bell peppers, pepper, salt, and carrot, and cook for 10 minutes. Set another pan over high heat, add in duck slices and cook each side for 3 minutes. Pour the mixture into the vegetable pan. Cook for 3 minutes. Serve.

Per serving: Cal 433; Net Carbs 8g; Fat 21g, Protein 53g

Herby Chicken Stew

Ingredients for 6 servings

2 tbsp butter

2 shallots, finely chopped

2 garlic cloves, minced

1 cup chicken broth

1 tsp dried rosemary

1 tsp dried thyme

1 lb chicken breasts, cubed

1 celery, chopped

1 carrot, chopped

1 bay leaf

1 chili pepper, chopped

2 tomatoes, chopped

Salt black pepper to taste

½ tsp paprika

Directions and Total Time: approx. 60 minutes

Melt butter in a pot over medium heat. Add in shallots, garlic, celery, carrot, salt, and pepper and sauté until tender, about 5 minutes. Pour in chicken broth, rosemary, thyme, chicken breasts, bay leaf, tomatoes, paprika, and chili pepper; bring to a boil. Reduce the heat to low. Simmer for 50 minutes. Discard the bay leaf and adjust the seasoning. Serve warm.

Per serving: Cal 240; Net Carbs 5g; Fat 9.6g, Protein 245

South-American Shrimp Stew

Ingredients for 6 servings

1 cup coconut milk

2 tbsp lime juice

¼ cup diced roasted peppers

1 ½ lb shrimp, deveined

¼ cup olive oil

1 garlic clove, minced

14 ounces diced tomatoes

2 tbsp sriracha sauce

¼ cup chopped onions

¼ cup chopped cilantro

Fresh dill, chopped to garnish

Salt and black pepper to taste

Directions and Total Time: approx. 25 minutes

Heat olive oil in a pot and add cook onions and garlic for 3 minutes. Add in tomatoes, shrimp, and cilantro. Cook for about 3-4 minutes. Stir in sriracha and coconut milk, and cook for 2 more minutes. Do not bring to a boil. Stir in lime juice and season with salt and pepper. Spoon the stew in bowls, garnish with fresh dill, and serve.

Per serving: Cal 324; Net Carbs 5g; Fat 21g, Protein
23g

Poultry

Chicken with Sour Cream Sauce

Preparation time: 10 minutes

Cooking time: 40 minutes

Servings: 4

Ingredients:

- chicken thighs
- Salt and ground black pepper, to taste
- 1 teaspoon onion powder
- ¼ cup sour cream
- 2 tablespoons sweet paprika

Directions:

Take a small bowl and mix onion powder, salt, pepper and paprika in it. Rub the paprika mixture over the chicken pieces. Place on a lined baking sheet. Bake in the oven at 400ºF for 45 minutes. Divide the chicken on a plate and set aside. Pour the pan juices into a mixing bowl and add the sour cream. Stir the sauce well and drizzle over the chicken.

Nutritional Value: Calories – 526, Fat – 22.4, Fiber – 1.3, Carbs – 2.5, Protein – 74.9

Rosemary Chicken with Avocado Sauce

Ingredients for 2 servings

Sauce

¼ cup mayonnaise

1 avocado, pitted

1 tbsp lemon juice

Salt to taste

Chicken

2 tbsp olive oil

2 chicken breasts

Salt and black pepper to taste

½ cup rosemary, chopped

Directions and Total Time: approx. 35 minutes

Take a bowl and mash the avocado with a fork. Add salt, mayonnaise and lemon juice and stir to combine. Take a pan and heat olive oil on medium heat. Season the chicken with pepper and salt and fry for 5 minutes and remove the chicken to a plate. Add rosemary and 1/4 cup water to the same pan. After boiling, reduce the heat and simmer for another 5 minutes. Add the chicken and cook covered for 10-15 minutes. Place chicken on a plate and serve with avocado sauce on the side.

Per serving: Cal 406; Net Carbs 3.9g; Fat 34g; Protein 22g

Chicken Stroganoff

Preparation time: 10 minutes

Cooking time: 4 hours and 10 minutes

Servings: 4

Ingredients:

- 2 garlic cloves, peeled and minced
- ounces mushrooms, chopped
- ¼ teaspoon celery seeds, ground
- 1 cup chicken stock
- 1 cup coconut milk
- 1 onion, peeled and chopped
- 1 pound chicken breasts, cut into medium–sized pieces
- 1½ teaspoons dried thyme
- 2 tablespoons fresh parsley, chopped
- Salt and ground black pepper, to taste
- zucchini, cut with a spiralizer

Directions:

Place the chicken in a slow cooker and add thyme, half of the parsley, salt, pepper, ginger, mushrooms, coconut milk, stock, celery seeds. Stir and cover to cook for 4 hours. Take a pan, heat water on medium temperature, add some salt and bring it to a boil. Then add the zucchini pasta, cook for 1 minute and drain. Divide between plates and serve with chicken mixture on top.

Nutritional Value: Calories – 413, Fat – 23.4, Fiber – 4.7, Carbs – 15.1, Protein – 38.9

Stuffed Chicken Breasts

Ingredients for 2 servings

2 tbsp butter

2 chicken breasts

1 cup baby spinach

1 carrot, shredded

1 tomato, chopped

¼ cup goat cheese

Salt and black pepper to taste

1 tsp dried oregano

2 cucumbers, spiralized

2 tbsp olive oil

1 tbsp rice vinegar

1 tbsp fresh dill, chopped

Directions and Total Time: approx. 60 minutes

First preheat the oven to 390 F. Grease a baking dish with cooking spray. Melt half the butter in a pan over medium heat and sauté the carrots, spinach and tomatoes for 5 minutes until soft. Sprinkle salt and pepper over it. Take a medium bowl and stir in it and let it cool for 10 minutes. Stir in oregano and goat cheese and set aside. Cut chicken breast and fill with cheese mixture. Set in a baking dish. Sprinkle with salt and pepper and brush with remaining butter. Bake for 30 minutes until done. Arrange the cucumbers neatly on a serving plate and coat with salt, pepper, vinegar and olive oil. Serve with stuffed chicken.

Per serving: Cal 861; Net Carbs 9.5g; Fat 58g; Protein 67g

Chicken Gumbo

Preparation time: 10 minutes

Cooking time: 7 hours

Servings: 5

Ingredients:

* 2 sausages, sliced
* chicken breasts, cubed
* 2 tablespoons dried oregano
* 2 bell peppers, seeded and chopped
* 1 onion, peeled and chopped
* 28 ounces canned diced tomatoes
* tablespoons dried thyme
* 2 tablespoons garlic powder
* 2 tablespoons dry mustard
* 1 teaspoon cayenne powder
* 1 tablespoons chili powder
* Salt and ground black pepper, to taste
* tablespoons Creole seasoning

Directions:

Take a slow cooker and add creole seasoning, chilli, red pepper, tomato, garlic powder, dry mustard, thyme, onion, oregano, salt, pepper, bell pepper and mix the sausage. Cover and cook on low flame for 7 hours. Open the lid of the slow cooker and stir and divide into bowls. Serve hot.

Nutritional Value: Calories – 445, Fat – 20.7, Fiber – 3.8, Carbs – 13, Protein – 50.9

Turnip Greens & Artichoke Chicken

Ingredients for 4 servings

4 oz canned artichoke hearts, chopped

4 oz cream cheese

2 chicken breasts, sliced

1 cup turnip greens

¼ cup Pecorino cheese, grated

½ tbsp onion powder

½ tbsp garlic powder

Salt and black pepper to taste

2 oz Monterrey Jack, shredded

Directions and Total Time: approx. 40 minutes

Line a baking sheet with parchment paper and arrange the chicken pieces. Sprinkle with salt and pepper and bake in the oven at 350 F for 25 minutes. Take a bowl and mix the rest of the ingredients well. Remove the chicken from the oven and spread over the artichokes, top with Monterey cheese, bake for another 5 minutes and serve hot.

Per serving: Cal 473; Net Carbs 6.2g; Fat 29g; Protein 41g

Chicken Thighs with Mushrooms and Cheese

Preparation time: 10 minutes

Cooking time: 45 minutes

Servings: 4

Ingredients:

- tablespoons butter
- ounces mushrooms, sliced
- 2 tablespoons gruyere cheese, grated
- Salt and ground black pepper, to taste
- 2 garlic cloves, peeled and minced
- chicken thighs

Directions:

Take a pan and heat 1 tablespoon of butter in it on medium flame. Add chicken thighs and sprinkle with salt and pepper. Cook on each side and remove to a baking dish. Reheat the pan over medium heat with the remaining butter, add the garlic and mushrooms, stir and cook for 1 minute. Add salt and pepper and cook for 10 minutes. Spoon mixture over chicken, sprinkle with cheese, and bake in oven at 350 F for 30 minutes. Turn on the oven broiler and broil everything for 2 minutes. Divide into plates and serve.

Nutritional Value: Calories – 729, Fat – 34.2, Fiber – 0.6, Carbs – 2.4, Protein – 98

Cheesy Pinwheels with Chicken

Ingredients for 4 servings

2 tbsp ghee 1 garlic clove, minced

1/3 lb chicken breasts, cubed

1 tsp creole seasoning

1/3 red onion, chopped

1 tomato, chopped

½ cup chicken stock

¼ cup whipping cream

½ cup mozzarella, grated

¼ cup fresh cilantro, chopped

Salt and black pepper to taste

4 oz cream cheese

5 eggs

A pinch of garlic powder

Directions and Total Time: approx. 40 minutes

Season chicken with creole seasoning. Take a kadai and heat 1 tbsp ghee in it on medium heat. Add chicken to that kadai and cook it on each side and take it out in a plate. Add the garlic and tomatoes to the remaining ghee. Cook for 5 minutes. Return the chicken to the pan and add the stock and cook for 15 minutes. Add red onion, salt, mozzarella cheese, whipping cream and black pepper and cook for 3 minutes. Place the mixture on a lined baking sheet. and bake in a preheated oven at 320 F for 10 minutes. After the cheese has cooled, place it on a cutting board. Roll and cut into medium slices. Place the slices neatly on a plate. Spread the chicken mixture on it. Sprinkle coriander before serving.

Per serving: Cal 363; Net Carbs 6.3g; Fat 28g; Protein 20g

Pecan-crusted Chicken

Preparation time: 10 minutes

Cooking time: 20 minutes

Servings: 4

Ingredients:

- 1 egg, whisked
- Salt and ground black pepper, to taste
- tablespoons coconut oil
- 1½ cups pecans, chopped
- chicken breasts

Directions:

Take two bowls, put the pecans in one and the beaten egg in the other. Dip seasoned chicken in egg and then dip in pecans. Heat oil in a pan on medium heat. Add chicken to it and cook it on both sides. Place the chicken pieces on a baking sheet and place in the oven. Bake at 350 F for 10 minutes. Divide between plates and serve.

Nutritional Value: Calories – 930, Fat – 65.2, Fiber – 5.3, Carbs – 7.1, Protein – 80.6

Thyme Chicken with Mushrooms & Turnip

Ingredients for 4 servings

3 cups mixed mushrooms, teared up

2 tbsp olive oil

4 tbsp butter, melted

1 lb chicken breasts, sliced

4 tbsp white wine

1 turnip, sliced

2 cloves garlic, minced

4 sprigs thyme, chopped

1 lemon, juiced

Salt and black pepper to taste

2 tbsp Dijon mustard

Directions and Total Time: approx. 50 minutes

Preheat the oven to 420 F. Place the turnips on a baking sheet, add a little oil and bake for 15 minutes. Take a bowl and mix roasted turnip, chicken, lemon juice, salt, pepper and mustard, garlic, mushroom, thyme evenly. Divide the chicken mixture between 4 large pieces of aluminum foil. Drizzle with olive oil, white wine and butter. Seal the edges to form a packet and place on a baking tray and bake for 25 minutes and serve hot.

Per serving: Cal 394; Net Carbs 4.6g; Fat 29g; Protein 25g

Pepperoni Chicken Bake

- Preparation time: 10 minutes
- Cooking time: 55 minutes
- Servings: 6

Ingredients:

- 14 ounces tomato passata
- 1 tablespoon coconut oil
- medium chicken breasts, skinless and boneless
- Salt and ground black pepper, to taste
- 1 teaspoon dried oregano

- ounces mozzarella cheese, sliced
- 1 teaspoon garlic powder
- 2 ounces pepperoni, sliced

Directions:

Take a saucepan and put tomato paste in it, bring it to a boil on medium heat and boil for 4 minutes and switch off the heat. Take a bowl and mix salt, pepper, chicken, oregano and garlic powder in it and stir. Heat coconut oil in a pan on medium heat. Add the chicken pieces and cook on each side and place in a baking dish. Spread mozzarella cheese slice on top. Add pepperoni slice on top. Bake for 30 minutes with oven set to 400 F. Divide between plates and serve.

Nutritional Value: Calories – 491, Fat – 24.4, Fiber – 0.2, Carbs – 4.7, Protein – 60.3

Fried Chicken

Preparation time: 24 hours

Cooking time: 20 minutes

Servings: 4

Ingredients:

- chicken breasts, cut into strips
- ounces pork rinds, crushed
- 2 cups coconut oil
- 16 ounces jarred pickle juice
- 2 eggs, whisked

Directions:

Take a bowl, mix the chicken breast pieces with butter juice, stir a little and cover it. Keep in refrigerator for 24 hours. Take two bowls and put eggs in one and pork in the other. Dip the chicken pieces in the egg and then coat the pork pieces well. Take a pan and heat oil on medium heat, add chicken pieces and fry for 3-4 minutes on each side. Transfer to a paper towel to drain the grease and serve.

Nutritional Value: Calories – 1488, Fat – 134.8, Fiber – 0, Carbs – 2.4, Protein – 73.8

Green Bean & Broccoli Chicken Stir-Fry

Ingredients for 2 servings

2 chicken breasts, cut into strips

2 tbsp olive oil

1 tsp red pepper flakes

1 tsp onion powder

1 tbsp fresh ginger, grated

¼ cup tamari sauce

½ tsp garlic powder

½ cup water

½ cup xylitol

4 oz green beans, chopped

½ tsp xanthan gum

½ cup green onions, chopped

10 oz broccoli florets

Directions and Total Time: approx. 45 minutes

Steam broccoli and green beans for 5 minutes until crisp and set aside. Take a pan and heat olive oil on medium heat. Add chicken and ginger to it and cook for 5 minutes. Add the rest of the ingredients and stir and cook for 15 minutes. Stir in the broccoli and peas and cook for 5 minutes and serve.

Per serving: Cal 411; Net Carbs 6.2g; Fat 25g; Protein 28g

Chicken Calzone

Preparation time: 10 minutes

Cooking time: 1 hour

Servings: 12

Ingredient s :

- 2 eggs
- ½ cup Parmesan cheese, grated
- 1 pound chicken breasts, skinless, boneless, and each sliced in half
- ½ cup marinara sauce
- 1 teaspoon Italian seasoning
- 1 teaspoon onion powder
- 1 teaspoon garlic powder
- Salt and ground black pepper, to taste
- ¼ cup flaxseed, ground
- ounces provolone cheese
- For pizza crust:
- eggs
- oz. shredded mozzarella

Directions:

Take a bowl and mix garlic powder, Italian seasoning onion powder, salt, pepper, flaxseed and parmesan cheese and mix well. In the second one, add a pinch of salt and pepper to the egg and beat it. Dip the chicken pieces in the egg and then place all the pieces in the spice mixture on a lined baking sheet. and bake in the oven at 350 F for 30 minutes. For the pizza crust, take a bowl and crack eggs, add cheese and mix well. Spread the mixture on a baking sheet lined with parchment paper. Bake at 350 F for 5 minutes. Place pizza crust on a lined baking sheet and spread provolone cheese over half. Remove the chicken from the oven, shred it and spread it over the provolone cheese. Add the marinara sauce and then the rest of the sauce. Shape half of the dough into a calzone. Seal the edges and place in the oven with the oven set to 350 F and bake for 20 minutes. Let the calzone cool before serving.

Nutritional Value: Calories – 247, Fat – 14.9, Fiber – 0.7, Carbs – 2.4, Protein – 25.2

Zucchini & Bell Pepper Chicken Gratin

Ingredients for 2 servings

1 red bell pepper, sliced

1 zucchini, chopped

Salt and black pepper to taste

1 tsp garlic powder

1 tbsp olive oil

2 chicken breasts, sliced

1 tomato, chopped

½ tsp dried oregano

½ tsp dried basil

½ cup mozzarella, shredded

Directions and Total Time: approx. 40 minutes

Coat the chicken with garlic powder, black pepper and salt. Heat olive oil in a pan on medium heat and add chicken pieces. Cook and take out in a baking dish. In the same pan, add bell peppers, tomatoes, zucchini, basil, salt and oregano and cook for 3 minutes. Spread the mixture over the chicken. Bake in the oven at 360 F for 20 minutes. Sprinkle the mozzarella over the chicken and serve.

Per serving: Cal 397; Net Carbs 6.2g; Fat 23g; Protein 45g

Mexican Chicken Soup

Preparation time: 10 minutes

Cooking time: 4 hours

Servings: 6

Ingredients:

- 1½ pounds chicken tights, skinless, boneless, and cubed
- 15 ounces chicken stock
- 15 ounces tomato passata
- ounces Monterey jack

Directions:

Mix cheese, tomato paste, chicken in slow cooker, stir and cover and cook for 4 hours. Divide into bowls and serve.

Nutritional Value: Calories – 397, Fat – 27.7, Fiber – 0, Carbs – 4.2, Protein – 34.4

Marinated Fried Chicken

Ingredients for 2 servings

2 tbsp olive oil

2 chicken breasts, cut into strips

½ cup pork rinds, crushed

8 oz jarred pickle juice

1 egg

Directions and Total Time: approx. 15 min + cooling time

Place the chicken in a bowl, cover with pickle juice and refrigerate for 12 hours. Place the pork in a bowl and beat the eggs in a bowl. Dip the chicken and pork pieces in the egg, making sure they are well coated. Heat olive oil in a pan over medium heat. Fry chicken on each side and drain on paper towels. Serve hot.

Per serving: Cal 489; Net Carbs 2g; Fat 46g; Protein 45g

Simple Chicken Stir-fry

Preparation time: 10 minutes

Cooking time: 12 minutes

Servings: 2

Ingredients:

- chicken thighs, skinless, boneless, and cut into thin strips
- 1 tablespoon sesame oil
- 1 teaspoon red pepper flakes
- 1 teaspoon onion powder
- 1 tablespoon fresh ginger, grated
- ¼ cup tamari sauce
- ½ teaspoon garlic powder
- ½ cup water
- 1 tablespoon stevia
- ½ teaspoon xanthan gum
- ½ cup scallions, chopped
- 2 cups broccoli florets

Directions :

Heat oil in a pan on medium heat, add chicken and ginger and cook for 5 minutes, stirring. Mix onion powder, water, tamari sauce, garlic powder, stevia, pepper flakes, xanthan gum and cook for 5 minutes. Add the scallions and broccoli and cook for 3 minutes, stirring. Divide between plates and serve hot.

Nutritional Value: Calories – 392, Fat – 19.1, Fiber – 3.6, Carbs – 11.3, Protein – 43.9

Mediterranean Stuffed Chicken Breasts

Ingredients for 4 servings

1 tbsp olive oil

1 cup spinach, chopped

2 chicken breasts Salt and black pepper to taste

½ cup cream cheese, softened

½ cup goat cheese, crumbled

1 garlic clove, minced

½ cup white wine

1 tbsp rosemary, chopped

Directions and Total Time: approx. 35 minutes

Take half a cup of water and add spinach to it and wilt it in a saucepan. Combine garlic, salt, goat cheese, cream cheese and pepper in a bowl and mix. Slice each chicken breast and stuff it with the spinach mixture. Take a pan and heat oil on medium heat. Add the stuffed chicken and cook for 5 minutes on each side. Transfer to a greased baking tray. Deglaze with white wine and 2 tablespoons water. Place in the oven and bake for 20 minutes. Once done, cut in half and serve sprinkled with rosemary.

Per serving: Cal 455; Net Carbs 2g; Fat 32g; Protein 37g

Spinach and Artichoke Chicken

Preparation time: 10 minutes

Cooking time: 50 minutes

Servings: 4

Ingredients:

- ounces cream cheese
- chicken breasts
- ounces canned artichoke hearts, chopped
- ounces spinach
- ½ cup Parmesan cheese, grated
- 1 tablespoon onion powder
- 1 tablespoon garlic powder
- Salt and ground black pepper, to taste
- ounces mozzarella cheese, shredded

Directions:

Place the chicken breasts on a lined baking sheet. Sprinkle with salt and pepper and place in the oven at 400 F and bake for 25 minutes. Take a bowl and mix garlic, salt, pepper, parmesan cheese, spinach, cream cheese, onion and artichoke. Remove the chicken from the oven. And cut each piece in half. Divide artichoke mixture, sprinkle with mozzarella cheese. Bake in the oven at 400 F for 20 minutes and serve hot.

Nutritional Value: Calories – 573, Fat – 30.6, Fiber – 5.4, Carbs – 12.5, Protein – 63.5

Pancetta & Cheese Stuffed Chicken

Ingredients for 2 servings

4 slices pancetta

2 tbsp olive oil

2 chicken breasts

1 garlic clove, minced

1 shallot, finely chopped

2 tbsp dried oregano

4 oz mascarpone cheese

1 lemon, zested

Salt and black pepper to taste

Directions and Total Time: approx. 35 minutes

Take a small pan, heat oil in it and saute garlic and mussels for 5 minutes. Mix pepper, salt and lemon juice in it. Take a bowl and transfer it to it and keep it to cool. Stir in oregano and mascarpone cheese. Cut into chicken breasts and fill with cheese mixture. Wrap each breast with 2 slices of pancetta and secure the ends with toothpicks. Place the chicken on a greased baking sheet. Cook in the oven at 380 F for 20 minutes and serve hot.

Per serving: Cal 636; Net Carbs 8.2g; Fat 45g; Protein 45g

Chicken Meatloaf

Cooking time: 40 minutes

Servings: 8

Preparation time: 10 minutes

Ingredients:

- 1 cup tomato sauce
- 1 teaspoon minced garlic
- 1 teaspoon dried basil
- 1/2 teaspoon dried rosemary
- pound ground chicken
- 2 tablespoons fresh parsley, chopped
- garlic cloves, peeled and minced
- 2 teaspoons onion powder
- 2 teaspoons Italian seasoning
- Salt and ground black pepper, to taste

- For the filling:
- ½ cup ricotta cheese
- 1 cup Parmesan cheese, grated
- 1 cup mozzarella cheese, shredded
- 2 teaspoons fresh chives, chopped
- 2 tablespoons fresh parsley, chopped
- 1 garlic clove, peeled and minced

Directions:

Take a bowl and mix garlic, basil, chicken half tomato paste, salt, pepper, rosemary, 3 garlic cloves, Italian seasoning, onion powder, 2 teaspoons of oats and stir. In another bowl, mix chives, half of mozzarella cheese, ricotta cheese, half of Parmesan cheese, half of mozzarella cheese, salt, pepper, 1 clove of garlic, 2 tablespoons of oats and stir. Place half of the chicken mix in the loaf pan and spread evenly. Add cheese filling. and spread evenly. Top with remaining meat and spread again. Place the meatloaf in the oven at 400 F and bake for 20 minutes. Remove meatloaf from oven, spread garlic, basil, tomato paste, rosemary, remaining cheese. and bake for 20 minutes. Let the meatloaf cool. Cut into pieces and serve on plates.

Nutritional Value: Calories – 334, Fat – 15.6, Fiber – 0.5, Carbs – 3.7, Protein – 43.9

Chicken Breasts with Creamy Kale Sauce

Ingredients for 2 servings

2 chicken breasts

1 cup heavy cream

2 tbsp butter

Salt and black pepper to taste

1 cup kale 1 tsp fresh sage

Directions and Total Time: approx. 20 minutes

Sprinkle salt and pepper over the chicken. Melt a spoonful of butter in a pan and cook the chicken breast in it for 10 minutes, turning once. Remove to a plate and let it cool then cut into pieces. In the same pan add heavy cream and cook for 3 minutes. Place the chicken on a plate and drizzle the sauce over it. Serve.

Per serving: Cal 571; Net Carbs 2.1g; Fat 44g; Protein 33g

One-pot Roasted Chicken

- Preparation time: 10 minutes
- Cooking time: 40 minutes
- Servings: 12

Ingredients:

- 1 whole chicken
- ½ teaspoon onion powder
- ½ teaspoon garlic powder
- Salt and ground black pepper, to taste
- tablespoons coconut oil
- 1 teaspoon Italian seasoning
- 1½ cups chicken stock
- 2 teaspoons guar gum

Directions:

Season the chicken with garlic powder, Italian seasoning, salt, pepper, half the oil and onion powder. Pour the remaining half of the oil into the instant pot and add the chicken and cover the pot. Cook for 40 minutes on poultry mode. Take the chicken in a plate and keep aside. Set the instant pot to saute mode and add the guar gum and stir and cook until thickened. Drizzle the sauce over the chicken and serve.

Nutritional Value: Calories – 463, Fat – 31.8, Fiber – 0, Carbs – 0.4, Protein – 44.1

Juicy Chicken with Broccoli & Pine Nuts

Ingredients for 4 servings

2 tbsp olive oil

2 chicken breasts, cut into strips

2 tbsp Worcestershire sauce

2 tsp balsamic vinegar

2 tsp xanthan gum

1 lemon, juiced

1 cup pine nuts

2 cups broccoli florets

1 onion, thinly sliced

Salt and black pepper to taste

1 tbsp cilantro, chopped

Directions and Total Time: approx. 25 minutes

Toast the pine nuts in a pan on medium heat for 2 minutes and keep aside. In the same pan, cook the olive oil until warm and the onion soft and remove the nuts. Take a bowl and mix balsamic vinegar, Worcestershire sauce, xanthan gum, lemon juice in it and keep it aside. Add chicken to the pan and cook for 5 minutes. Add black pepper and salt to the broccoli. Fry and add to the lemon mixture. Cook the sauce for 5 minutes and add the pine nuts and onion. Stir. Serve the chicken stir fry with coriander.

Per serving: Cal 386; Net Carbs 6.4g; Fat 30g; Protein 20g

Chicken with Green Onion Sauce

- Preparation time: 10 minutes
- Cooking time: 27 minutes
- Servings: 4

Ingredients:
- tablespoons butter
- 1 green onion, peeled and chopped
- chicken breast halves, skinless and boneless
- Salt and ground black pepper, to taste
- ounces sour cream

Directions:
Take a pan and heat it on medium high heat with butter. Add chicken pieces, salt and pepper to the pan and cover. Reduce heat and let simmer for 10 minutes. Open the covered pan and slice the chicken and cover and cook for another 10 minutes. Turn off the heat and add salt and pepper if needed. Add sour cream and stir well. Cover the pan and keep aside for 5 minutes. Stir well again and divide on plates and serve.
Nutritional Value: Calories – 659, Fat – 36.6, Fiber – 0.1, Carbs – 2.7, Protein – 75.8

Baked Chicken Nuggets

Ingredients for 2 servings
2 tbsp ranch dressing
½ cup almond flour
1 egg
2 tbsp garlic powder
2 chicken breasts, cubed
Salt and black pepper to taste
1 tbsp butter, melted

Directions and Total Time: approx. 30 minutes

Preheat the oven to 400 F. Grease a baking dish with butter. Take a bowl and mix together almond flour, garlic powder, salt and black pepper. Take another bowl and beat the egg in it. Dip the chicken cubes in the egg and then dip in the flour mixture and cook in the oven for 20 minutes. Drain on paper towels to remove excess grease. and serve with ranch dressing if desired.
Per serving: Cal 473; Net Carbs 7.6g; Fat 37g; Protein 31g

Chicken–stuffed Mushrooms

Preparation time: 10 minutes
Cooking time: 10 minutes
Servings: 6
Ingredients:
- ounces button mushroom caps
- ounces cream cheese
- ¼ cup butternut squash, chopped
- 1 teaspoon plain yogurt
- tablespoons hot sauce
- ¾ cup blue cheese, crumbled
- ¼ cup onion, chopped
- ½ cup chicken meat, already cooked and chopped
- Salt and ground black pepper, to taste
- Vegetable oil cooking spray

Directions:
Take a bowl and mix curd, salt, pepper, chicken, hot

sauce, squash, cream cheese, blue cheese and onion. Fill each mushroom cap with mixture, and place on a lined baking sheet. Spray with cooking spray and place in oven at 425 F and bake for 15 minutes. Divide between plates and serve.

Nutritional Value: Calories – 167, Fat – 12.4, Fiber – 0.9, Carbs – 4.3, Protein – 10.6

Peanut-Crusted Chicken

Ingredients for 4 servings

1 egg, beaten

Salt and black pepper to taste

3 tbsp canola oil

1 ½ cups ground peanuts

2 chicken breast halves

Lemon slices for garnish

Directions and Total Time: approx. 25 minutes

Sprinkle salt and pepper over the chicken. Dip in egg then dip in ground peanuts. Take a pan, heat the canola oil on medium heat and sear it on each side. Remove to a baking sheet. Place in a preheated 360 F oven and bake for 10 minutes. Serve with lemon wedges on top.

Per serving: Cal 654; Net Carbs 4.7g; Fat 52g; Protein 46g

Chicken–stuffed Avocados

Preparation time: 10 minutes

Cooking time: 0 minutes

Servings: 2

Ingredients:

- avocados, cut in half and pitted
- ¼ cup mayonnaise
- 1 teaspoon dried thyme
- 2 tablespoons cream cheese
- 1½ cups chicken, cooked and shredded
- Salt and ground black pepper, to taste
- ¼ teaspoon cayenne pepper
- ½ teaspoon onion powder
- ½ teaspoon garlic powder

- 1 teaspoon paprika
- 2 tablespoons lemon juice

Directions:

Scoop the inside of an avocado half and place the flesh in a bowl. Add the chicken to the avocado flesh and stir well. Add red pepper, salt, pepper, lemon juice, onion, garlic, paprika, cream cheese, thyme, egg mixture and mix well. Serve stuffed with chicken mixture.

Nutritional Value: Calories – 1142, Fat – 64.2, Fiber – 13.7, Carbs – 24.9, Protein – 116.5

Chicken Dippers with Homemade Ketchup

Ingredients for 4 servings

1 lb chicken breasts, cut into strips

14 oz canned tomatoes, diced

1 tbsp tomato paste

½ tbsp xylitol

1 tbsp balsamic vinegar

1 cup tomato sauce

1 tbsp basil, chopped

½ cup almond flour

¼ cup Parmesan, grated

½ tsp garlic powder

1 tsp dried parsley

½ tsp dried thyme Salt

and black pepper to taste

1 egg, beaten in a bowl

2 tbsp olive oil

Directions and Total Time: approx. 35 minutes

Take a saucepan and heat it on medium heat. Add xylitol, tomato paste, tomatoes, salt, pepper, tomato sauce and balsamic vinegar and bring to a boil. Cook for 15 minutes, stirring until thickened. Top with ketchup and basil. Take a bowl and mix together the oats, almond flour, parmesan, pepper, garlic powder, thyme and salt. Dip the chicken in the egg and almond flour mixture. Heat olive oil in a pan over medium heat. After the chicken is fried, remove and serve with ketchup.

Per serving: Cal 336; Net Carbs 7.7g; Fat 21g; Protein 25g

Balsamic Chicken

Preparation time: 10 minutes
Cooking time: 20 minutes
Servings: 4

Ingredients:

- tablespoons coconut oil
- pounds chicken breasts, skinless and boneless
- garlic cloves, peeled and minced
- Salt and ground black pepper, to taste
- 1 cup chicken stock
- tablespoons stevia
- ½ cup balsamic vinegar
- 1 tomato, sliced thin
- mozzarella slices
- Fresh basil, chopped, for serving

Directions:

Take a pan and heat it with oil on medium high temperature. Add chicken pieces, salt, pepper and cook both sides and reduce the heat. Stir in the vinegar, garlic, stevia, stock and turn the heat up to high again and cook for 10 minutes. Place the chicken breasts on a lined baking sheet. Top with mozzarella cheese and basil. Bake in the oven until the cheese melts and place the tomato slices on top of the chicken pieces and serve between plates.

Nutritional Value: Calories – 654, Fat – 34.7, Fiber – 0.2, Carbs – 4.8, Protein – 78.1

Winter Chicken with Vegetables

Ingredients for 4 servings
2 tbsp olive oil
2 cups whipping cream
1 lb chicken breasts, chopped
1 onion, chopped
1 carrot, chopped
2 cups chicken stock
Salt and black pepper to taste

1 bay leaf
1 turnip, chopped
1 parsnip, chopped
1 cup green beans, chopped
2 tsp fresh thyme, chopped

Directions and Total Time: approx. 40 minutes

Heat oil in a pan on medium heat. Sauté the onion, add the stock, turnips, carrots, chicken, parsnips and bay leaves. Bring to a boil and let simmer for 20 minutes. Add peas and cook for 5 minutes. Stir in the whipping cream, discarding the bay leaf. and sprinkle with thyme to serve.

Per serving: Cal 513; Net Carbs 10g; Fat 32g; Protein 33g

Chicken Pasta

Preparation time: 10 minutes
Cooking time: 30 minutes
Servings: 4

Ingredients:

- tablespoons butter
- 1 teaspoon garlic, minced
- 1 pound chicken cutlets
- 1 teaspoon Cajun seasoning
- ¼ cup scallions, chopped
- ½ cup tomatoes, cored and chopped
- ½ cup chicken stock
- ¼ cup whipping cream
- ½ cup cheddar cheese, grated
- 1 ounce cream cheese
- ¼ cup fresh cilantro, chopped
- Salt and ground black pepper, to taste
- For the pasta:
- ounces cream cheese
- eggs
- Salt and ground black pepper, to taste
- A pinch of garlic powder

Directions:

Heat butter in a pan on medium heat. Add chicken

cutlet to it. Add Cajun seasoning and cook for 2 minutes. Remove in a plate. Heat over medium heat with remaining butter, add garlic, stir and cook for 2 minutes. Add tomatoes and cook for 2 minutes. Add stock and remaining Cajun seasoning and cook for 5 minutes. Stir in 1 ounce of cream cheese, salt, pepper, whipping cream, cheddar cheese, scallions, cilantro and turn off the heat. In a blender, mix eggs, salt, pepper, garlic powder, 4 ounces of cream cheese, and pulse well. Place on a lined baking dish and set aside for 5 minutes. and then bake in the oven at 325 F for 10 minutes. Divide the pasta between plates and serve with the chicken mixture on top.

Nutritional Value: Calories – 602, Fat – 42.4, Fiber – 0.5, Carbs – 3.5, Protein – 50.7

Chicken Kabobs with Celery Root Chips

Ingredients for 2 servings

4 tbsp olive oil

2 chicken breasts, cubed

Salt and black pepper to taste

1 tsp dried oregano

1 tsp chili powder

¼ cup chicken broth

1 lb celery root, sliced

Directions and Total Time: approx. 60 minutes

Preheat the oven to 400 F. Take a large bowl and mix the oregano, olive oil, half the oil, salt, pepper, cumin and add the chicken. Toss to coat and refrigerate for 15 minutes. Arrange the celery slices on a greased baking tray and drizzle with the remaining olive oil. Sprinkle with salt and pepper. Bake for 10 minutes. Take the chicken from the refrigerator and thread it onto skewers. Serve.

Per serving: Cal 565; Net Carbs 5.6g; Fat 43g; Protein 35

Peanut–grilled Chicken

Preparation time: 10 minutes

Cooking time: 20 minutes

Servings: 8

Ingredients:

- 2½ pounds chicken thighs, and drumsticks
- 1 tablespoon coconut aminos
- 1 tablespoon apple cider vinegar
- A pinch of red pepper flakes
- Salt and ground black pepper, to taste
- ½ teaspoon ground ginger
- ⅓ cup peanut butter
- 1 garlic clove, peeled and minced
- ½ cup warm water

Directions:

Mix water, peanut butter, salt, pepper, amino, ginger, pepper flakes, garlic, vinegar well in a blender. Pat the chicken pieces dry and add the peanut butter marinade to the pan. Toss to coat and refrigerate for 1 hour. Place the chicken pieces on a preheated pan over medium heat, flip and cook for 10 minutes. Brush with some marinade and cook for 10 minutes. Divide on plates and serve.

Nutritional Value: Calories – 1196, Fat – 49.5, Fiber – 0.7, Carbs – 2.4, Protein – 174.9

Pork

Pancetta & Egg Plate with Cherry Tomatoes

Ingredients for 4 servings

5 oz pancetta, chopped

2 tbsp olive oil

8 eggs

1 tbsp butter, softened

¼ cup cherry tomatoes, halved

2 tbsp chopped oregano

Directions and Total Time: approx. 30 minutes

Take a kadai and heat half oil on medium heat. Fry pancetta until crisp and set aside. Heat olive oil in a pan and crack 4 eggs. Cook until the whites set, but the yolks are still runny, 1 minute. Spoon two eggs onto two plates next to the pancetta and fry the remaining eggs with the remaining oil. Melt the butter in a pan, fry the tomatoes until the edges turn brown. Garnish with oregano and serve.

Per serving: Cal 278; Net Carbs 0.5g; Fat 23g; Protein 20g

Chorizo in Cabbage Sauce with Pine Nuts

Ingredients for 4 servings

25 oz green canon cabbage, shredded

6 tbsp butter

25 oz chorizo sausages

1 ¼ cups coconut cream

½ cup fresh sage, chopped

½ lemon, zested

2 tbsp toasted pine nuts

Directions and Total Time: approx. 30 minutes

Take a pan, melt 2 tablespoons of butter in it and fry the chorizo for 10 minutes until it turns brown on the outside. Remove in a plate. Melt the remaining butter and saute the cabbage. Mix in the coconut cream and simmer until the cream reduces. Season with sage, salt, pepper, and lemon zest. Divide the chorizo between 4 plates and spoon each plate aside and sprinkle with pine nuts. And serve hot.

Per serving: Cal 914; Net Carbs 16.9g; Fat 76g; Protein 38g

Hawaiian Pork Loco Moco

Ingredients for 4 servings

1 ½ lb ground pork

1/3 cup flaxseed meal

½ tsp nutmeg powder

1 tsp onion powder

5 large egg

2 tbsp heavy cream

3 tbsp coconut oil

1 tbsp salted butter

1 shallot, finely chopped

1 cup sliced oyster mushrooms

1 cup vegetable stock

1 tsp Worcestershire sauce

1 tsp tamari sauce

½ tsp xanthan gum

2 tbsp olive oil

4 large eggs

Directions and Total Time: approx. 40 minutes

Take a bowl and mix together salt, pepper, nutmeg, flaxseed meal, pork and onion powder. In another bowl, beat 1 egg with heavy cream and mix into the pork mixture. After the dough becomes sticky, mold 8 patties from the mixture and keep aside. Heat coconut oil in a pan. Fry the patties well on both sides and keep aside. Melt the butter in the same pan and cook the shallots and mushrooms for 5 minutes until soft. In a bowl, mix the tamari sauce, stock, Worcestershire, salt and pepper. Pour the mixture over the mushrooms and cook for 5 minutes. Stir in the xanthan gum. Heat half the olive oil in a pan. Crack the eggs and fry them. Fry the remaining eggs using the remaining olive oil. Serve pork with mushroom gravy.

Per serving: Cal 655; Net Carbs 2.2g; Fat 46g; Protein 55g

Pork Sausage Omelet with Mushrooms

Ingredients for 2 servings

¼ cup sliced cremini mushrooms

2 tbsp olive oil

2 oz pork sausage, crumbled

1 small white onion, chopped

2 tbsp butter

6 eggs

2 oz shredded cheddar cheese

Directions and Total Time: approx. 30 minutes

Heat olive oil in a pan on medium heat. Add the pork sausage and fry for 10 minutes and set aside. Saute the onion and mushroom in the same pan and keep aside. Melt the butter over low heat. Take a bowl and whisk eggs, salt and black pepper until smooth and frothy. Add eggs to pan and swirl to spread. When the omelet begins to firm up, top with the pork, mushroom onion mixture, and cheese. Using a spatula, carefully scrape the egg around the edges of the pan and flip over the stuffing for 2 minutes. Serve.

Per serving: Cal 534; Net Carbs 2.7g; Fat 43g; Protein 29g

British Pork Pie with Broccoli Topping

Ingredients for 4 servings

1 head broccoli, cut into florets

½ cup crème fraîche

1 whole egg

½ celery, finely chopped

3 oz butter, melted

5 oz shredded Swiss cheese

2 tbsp butter, cold

2 lb ground pork

2 tbsp tamari sauce

2 tbsp Worcestershire sauce

½ tbsp hot sauce

1 tsp onion powder

Directions and Total Time: approx. 55 minutes

Preheat the oven to 400 F. Boil salted water in a pot and cook the broccoli for 5 minutes. Drain and transfer to a food processor. Grind until it becomes like rice. Drain the broccoli into a bowl. Add eggs, celery, crème fraîche, butter, half the Swiss cheese, salt and pepper. Mix until evenly combined. Take a pot, melt cold butter in it, add pork and cook for 10 minutes. Mix onion powder, tamari, Worcestershire sauce, salt and pepper. Spread in a greased baking dish and cover with the broccoli mixture. Sprinkle with remaining cheese and bake for 20 minutes. Serve with greens.

Per serving: Cal 701; Net Carbs 3.3g; Fat 49g; Protein 60g

Hot Tex-Mex Pork Casserole

Ingredients for 4 servings

2 tbsp butter

1 ½ lb ground pork

3 tbsp Tex-Mex seasoning

2 tbsp chopped jalapeños

½ cup crushed tomatoes

½ cup shredded Monterey Jack

1 scallion, chopped to garnish

1 cup sour cream, for serving

Directions and Total Time: approx. 40 minutes

Preheat the oven to 330 F and grease a baking dish with cooking spray. Take a pan, melt the butter in it and cook the pork for 10 minutes. Stir in Tex-Mex seasoning, jalapeños, and tomatoes; Simmer for 5 minutes and season to taste. Remove the mixture to a dish. Sprinkle cheese on top and bake for 20 minutes until cheese is browned. Serve garnished with sour cream and scallions.

Per serving: Cal 431; Net Carbs 7.8g; Fat 24g; Protein 43g

Thyme Pork Roast with Brussels Sprouts

Ingredients for 4 servings

2 lb pork roast

Salt and black pepper to taste

2 tsp dried thyme

1 bay leaf

5 black peppercorns

2 ½ cups beef broth

2 garlic cloves, minced

1 ½ oz fresh ginger, grated

1 tbsp coconut oil

1 tbsp smoked paprika

½ lb Brussel sprouts, halved

1 ½ cups coconut cream

Directions and Total Time: approx. 2 hours

Preheat the oven to 360 F. Place the meat in a deep baking dish and season with thyme, salt, pepper and bay leaf. Top with gravy and cover with aluminum foil. Bake for 90 minutes. Remove the foil and place the pork on a cutting board. Pour the juice into a bowl and cover. Combine coconut oil, garlic, ginger and paprika in a bowl. Apply the mixture over the meat. Roast for 10 minutes. Remove and cut into fine pieces and keep aside. Meanwhile, strain the juice through a sieve into a pot and boil until reduced to 1 ½ cups. Add in the Brussels sprouts and cook for 10 minutes until tender. Stir in the coconut cream and simmer for 10 minutes. Serve with Creamy Brussels Sprouts Roast Pork.

Per serving: Cal 691; Net Carbs 9.6g; Fat 45g; Protein 59g

Cheesy Pork Quiche

Ingredients for 4 servings

1 ¼ cups almond flour

1 tbsp psyllium husk powder

4 tbsp chia seeds

2 tbsp melted butter

6 egg

1 tbsp butter

½ lb smoked pork shoulder

1 yellow onion, chopped

1 tsp dried thyme

Salt and black pepper to taste

1 cup coconut cream

¼ cup shredded Swiss cheese

Directions and Total Time: approx. 70 minutes

Preheat oven to 350 F. Grease a springform pan with cooking spray. and line with parchment paper. Keep aside. Take a food processor and add chia seeds, almond flour, psyllium husk, butter, 1/2 teaspoon salt and 1 egg. Mix until a thick dough is formed. Oil your hands and spread the batter on the bottom of a springform pan. Refrigerate while filling. Take a pan, melt the butter and cook the pork and onion for 10 minutes. Season with salt, pepper and thyme and stir well. Remove the piecrust from the fridge and pour over the pork and onions. Take a bowl and whisk half of the Swiss cheese, coconut cream and remaining egg in it. Add the mixture to the meat filling. Bake for 45 minutes until cheese is melted. Remove the pan, leave the lock and serve in slices.

Per serving: Cal 498; Net Carbs 4.6g; Fat 42g; Protein 24g

Parmesan & Pimiento Pork Meatballs

Ingredients for 4 servings

¼ cup chopped pimientos

1/3 cup mayonnaise

3 tbsp softened cream cheese

1 tsp paprika powder

1 pinch cayenne pepper

1 tbsp Dijon mustard

4 oz grated Parmesan cheese

1 ½ lb ground pork

1 large egg

2 tbsp olive oil, for frying

Directions and Total Time: approx. 30 minutes

Take a bowl and mix paprika, cream cheese, cayenne pepper, pimentos, mayo, mustard, parmesan, salt, pepper, pork, and eggs. Mix by hand to form big meatballs. Take a non stick kadai and heat olive oil in it. Fry the meatballs for 10 minutes. Transfer to a plate and serve on a bed of green salad.

Per serving: Cal 485; Net Carbs 6.8g; Fat 30g; Protein 47g

Pork Bake with Cottage Cheese & Olives

Ingredients for 4 servings

½ cup cottage cheese, crumbled

2 tbsp avocado oil

1 ½ lb ground pork

¼ cup sliced Kalamata olives

2 garlic cloves, minced

½ cup marinara sauce

1 ¼ cups heavy cream

Directions and Total Time: approx. 40 minutes

Preheat oven to 400 F. Grease a casserole dish with cooking spray. Take a pan, heat olive oil in it, add pork and cook for 10 minutes. Stir evenly and do not allow lumps to form. Spread the pork in the bottom of the casserole dish. Add garlic, cottage cheese and olives on it. Take a bowl and mix the heavy cream and marinara sauce in it and add the whole meat. Bake for 20 minutes and serve hot.

Per serving: Cal 451; Net Carbs 1.5g; Fat 30g; Protein 40g

Buttered Pork Chops with Lemon Asparagus

Ingredients for 4 servings

7 tbsp butter

4 pork chops

Salt and black pepper to taste

4 tbsp butter, softened

2 garlic cloves, minced

1 lb asparagus, trimmed

1 tbsp dried cilantro

1 small lemon, juice

Directions and Total Time: approx. 30 minutes

Take a pan and melt 4 tablespoons of butter on medium heat. Sprinkle the pork with salt and pepper. Fry for 10 minutes on both sides and keep aside. Melt the remaining butter in a pan and fry the garlic in it. Add the asparagus and cook for 5 minutes until soft. Add coriander and lemon juice and coat well. Serve with pork chops and asparagus.

Per serving: Cal 538; Net Carbs 1.2g; Fat 38g; Protein 42g

Tasty Pork Chops with Cauliflower Steaks

Ingredients for 4 servings

2 heads cauliflower, cut into 4 steaks

4 pork chops

1 tbsp mesquite seasoning

2 tbsp butter

2 tbsp olive oil

½ cup Parmesan cheese

Directions and Total Time: approx. 30 minutes

Season the pork with salt, pepper, and mesquite seasoning. Take a skillet, melt butter in it and fry the pork on both sides and keep aside. Heat the olive oil in a grill pan and cook the cauli steaks for 5 minutes. Sprinkle with parmesan to melt. Serve steaks with pork chops.

Per serving: Cal 429; Net Carbs 3.9g; Fat 23g; Protein 45g

Zucchini & Tomato Pork Omelet

Ingredients for 4 servings

3 zucchinis, halved lengthwise

4 tbsp olive oil

1 garlic clove, crushed

1 small plum tomato, diced

2 tbsp chopped scallions

1 tsp dried basil

1 tsp cumin powder

1 tsp smoked paprika

1 lb ground pork

3 large eggs, beaten

3 tsp crushed pork rinds

1/3 cup chopped cilantro

Directions and Total Time: approx. 50 minutes

Heat a grill to medium heat, place zucchini on top, drizzle with 1 tablespoon olive oil and broil for 5 minutes. Keep aside. Take a pan, heat 1 tbsp of olive oil and saute tomatoes, scallions and garlic for 10 minutes. Mix salt, paprika, cumin, basil. Add the pork and cook for 10 minutes. Spread the pork mixture over the grilled zucchini slices and flatten the mixture. Heat the remaining oil in the same pan and place the zucchini in it. Crack the egg over the zucchinis and cover the pan and cook for 5 minutes until set. Serve topped with pork rinds and a sprinkling of cilantro.

Per serving: Cal 332; Net Carbs 1.1g; Fat 22g; Protein 30g

Italian Pork with Capers

Ingredients for 4 servings

1 ½ lb thin cut pork chops, boneless

½ lemon, juiced + 1 lemon, sliced

Salt and black pepper to taste

1 tbsp avocado oil

3 tbsp butter

2 tbsp capers

1 cup beef broth

2 tbsp chopped parsley

Directions and Total Time: approx. 30 minutes

Heat the avocado oil in a pan and cook the pork chops for 15 minutes. Cover to set aside in a plate. Take a pan, melt butter in it and cook capers till hot. Stir for 5 minutes. Add the lemon juice and mutton stock and simmer until the sauce is reduced by half. Add the pork back and top with the lemon wedges and sprinkle with 1 tablespoon of the egg. Boil for 5 minutes. Garnish with eggs and creamy mashed cauliflower.

Per serving: Cal 341; Net Carbs 0.8g; Fat 18g; Protein 40g

Avocado & Green Bean Pork Sauté

Ingredients for 4 servings

4 tbsp avocado oil

4 pork shoulder chops

2 tbsp avocado oil

1 ½ cups green beans

2 large avocados, chopped

Salt and black pepper to taste

6 green onions, chopped

1 tbsp chopped parsley

Directions and Total Time: approx. 30 minutes

Heat oil in a pan, add pork, pepper and salt and fry for 10 minutes. Saute the green beans in the same pan for 10 minutes. Stir in half the onion and avocado for 3 minutes. Remove to plates and garnish with remaining onions and ova. Serve with pork chops.

Per serving: Cal 557; Net Carbs 1.9g; Fat 36g; Protein 43g

Savory Pork Tacos

Ingredients for 4 servings

2 tbsp olive oil

½ cup sliced yellow onion

2 lb pork shoulder

4 tbsp ras el hanout seasoning

Salt to taste

3 ½ cups beef broth

5 tbsp psyllium husk powder

1 ¼ cups almond flour

2 eggs, cracked into a bowl

2 tbsp butter, for frying

Directions and Total Time: approx. 7 hours

Take a pot, heat olive oil in it and saute onion for 5 minutes. Add the juice el hanout, salt and onion to the pork shoulder. Sear each side and cover with mutton gravy. Reduce the heat and cook until the pork is tender. Shred the pork with two forks and cook for 1 hour and set aside. Take a bowl and mix together almond flour, psyllium husk powder and 1 tsp salt.

Mix eggs and add 1 cup of water until a thick dough is formed. Cut the dough into 8 pieces. Grease a parchment paper with cooking spray and place a piece of dough on top. Cover with another parchment paper and using a rolling pin, flatten the dough into a circle. Repeat the same process for remaining dough balls. Melt a quarter of the butter in a pan and fry the flatbreads one at a time until lightly browned on both sides. Transfer to tortilla plates and serve.

Per serving: Cal 520; Net Carbs 3.8g; Fat 30g; Protein 50g

Yummy Spareribs in Béarnaise Sauce

Ingredients for 4 servings

3 tbsp butter, melted

4 egg yolks, beaten

2 tbsp chopped tarragon

2 tsp white wine vinegar

½ tsp onion powder

Salt and black pepper to taste

4 tbsp butter

2 lb spareribs, divided into 16

Directions and Total Time: approx. 30 minutes

Take a bowl and mix the butter and egg yolks in it until they are evenly mixed. Take another bowl and mix onion powder, tarragon, white wine vinegar in it. Mix the egg mixture and sprinkle with salt and pepper. Keep aside. Melt the butter in a pan on medium heat. Cook in butter on both sides until browned with crust, 10 minutes. Remove spareribs to plates and serve with béarnaise sauce on the side.

Per serving: Cal 878; Net Carbs 1g; Fat 78g; Protein 41g

Pork & Pecan in Camembert Bake

Ingredients for 4 servings

9 oz whole Camembert cheese

½ lb boneless pork chops, cut into small cubes

3 tbsp olive oil

2 oz pecans

1 garlic clove, minced

1 tbsp chopped parsley

Directions and Total Time: approx. 30 minutes

Preheat the oven to 400 F. While the cheese is still in its box, using a knife, score about a ¼-inch round on the top and sides and remove the top layer of skin. Place the cheese on a baking tray and melt in the oven for 10 minutes. Take a pan, heat olive oil in it, add black pepper, salt and fry the pork. Remove to a bowl and add the oats, pecans and garlic. Spoon the mixture over the cheese and bake for 10 minutes until the cheese is soft.

Per serving: Cal 452; Net Carbs 0.2g; Fat 38g; Protein 27g

Cheddar Pork Burrito Bowl

Ingredients for 4 servings

1 tbsp butter

1 lb ground pork

½ cup beef broth

4 tbsp taco seasoning

Salt and black pepper to taste

½ cup sharp cheddar, shredded

½ cup sour cream

¼ cup sliced black olives

1 avocado, cubed

¼ cup tomatoes, diced

1 green onion, sliced

1 tbsp fresh cilantro, chopped

Directions and Total Time: approx. 30 minutes

Melt the butter in a pan on medium heat. Cook the pork for 10 minutes. Season with salt, taco seasoning, pepper and broth and cook for 5 minutes. Stir in half the cheddar cheese to melt. Spoon into a bowl and top with olives, avocado, tomato, green onion and cilantro to serve.

Per serving: Cal 386; Net Carbs 8.8g; Fat 23g; Protein 30g

Parmesan Pork Stuffed Mushrooms

Ingredients for 4 servings

12 medium portabella mushrooms, stalks removed

2 tbsp butter

½ lb ground pork

1 tsp paprika

3 tbsp chives, finely chopped

7 oz cream cheese

¼ cup shredded Parmesan

Directions and Total Time: approx. 30 minutes

Preheat the oven to 400 F and grease a baking sheet with cooking spray. Take a pan, melt butter on medium heat, add salt, pepper, pork and paprika. Stir well for 10 minutes. Mix until the cream cheese and chives are evenly combined. Place the mushrooms on a baking sheet and spoon the mixture over them. Bake for 10 minutes until mushroom cheese melts. Remove in plates and serve.

Per serving: Cal 299; Net Carbs 2.2g; Fat 23g; Protein 19g

Florentine-Style Pizza with Bacon

Ingredients for 2 servings

1 cup shredded provolone cheese

1 (7 oz) can sliced mushrooms, drained

10 eggs

1 tsp Italian seasoning

6 bacon slices

2/3 cup tomato sauce

2 cups chopped kale, wilted

½ cup grated mozzarella

4 eggs

Olive oil for drizzling

Directions and Total Time: approx. 45 minutes

Preheat the oven to 400 F and line a baking pan with parchment paper. Take a bowl, crack 6 eggs and add Italian seasoning and provolone cheese. Spread the mixture on a pizza baking pan and bake for 20 minutes. Let cool. Set the temperature to 450 F. Fry the bacon in a pan until crisp. Remove to a plate, spread the tomato sauce over the crust and add the mozzarella and mushrooms. Bake in the oven for 15 minutes. Crack the remaining 4 eggs on top and cover the bacon. Bake for 2-3 minutes until the eggs are set and serve hot.

Per serving: Cal 1093; Net Carbs 6.1g; Fat 77g; Protein 69g

Cheesy Mushrooms & Bacon Lettuce Rolls

Ingredients for 4 servings

½ cup sliced cremini mushrooms

1 iceberg lettuce, leaves separated

8 bacon slices, chopped

2 tbsp olive oil

1 ½ lb ground pork

1 cup shredded cheddar

Directions and Total Time: approx. 30 minutes

Take a skillet and cook bacon in it over medium heat until crisp. Transfer to a paper-towel-lined plate. Heat 1 tbsp of olive oil in a pan and fry the mushrooms in it. Season with salt and pepper and cook until tender. Heat the remaining meat and cook the pork in it for 10 minutes. Top with bacon and mushrooms. Roll up and serve with mayo.

Per serving: Cal 630; Net Carbs 0.5g; Fat 45g; Protein 52g

Saucy Thai Pork Medallions

Ingredients for 4 servings

1 ½ pork tenderloin, sliced into ½ -inch medallions

6 tbsp butter

1 canon cabbage, shredded

Salt and black pepper to taste

1 celery, chopped

1 tbsp red curry powder

1 ¼ cups coconut cream

Directions and Total Time: approx. 45 minutes

Melt 2 tbsp of butter in a pan and saute the cabbage until soft and keep aside. Melt 2 tablespoons of butter in a pan, add the pork, season with salt and pepper and fry and set aside. Add the remaining butter to the pan and saute the celery till soft. Mix in the curry and stir in the coconut cream. Serve with buttered cabbage.

Per serving: Cal 626; Net Carbs 3.9g; Fat 48g; Protein 43g

Barbecue Baked Pork Chops

Ingredients for 4 servings

½ cup grated flaxseed meal

1 tsp dried thyme

1 tsp paprika

Salt and black pepper to taste

¼ tsp chili powder

1 ½ tsp garlic powder

1 tbsp dried parsley

1/2 tsp onion powder

1/8 tsp basil

4 pork chops

1 tbsp melted butter

½ cup BBQ sauce

Directions and Total Time: approx. 70 minutes

Preheat the oven to 400 F. Take a bowl and mix thyme, salt, pepper, paprika, flaxseed meal, garlic powder, chilli, ova, basil and onion powder in it. Rub the pork chops with the mixture. Melt butter in a skillet and sear pork on both sides, 10 minutes. Transfer to a greased baking sheet, baste with BBQ sauce and bake for 50 minutes. Slice and serve with buttered parsnips.

Per serving: Cal 385; Net Carbs 1.6g; Fat 19g; Protein 44g

Dijon Pork Loin Roast

Ingredients for 6 servings

3 lb boneless pork loin roast

5 cloves garlic, minced

Salt and black pepper to taste

1 tbsp Dijon mustard

1 tsp dried basil

2 tsp garlic powder

Directions and Total Time: approx. 30 minutes

Preheat the oven to 400 F and place the pork in a baking dish. Take a bowl and mix salt, pepper, mustard, basil, chopped garlic and garlic powder in it. Spread the mixture over the pork. Drizzle with olive oil and bake for 20 minutes. Remove and cool. Serve sliced with greens.

Per serving: Cal 311; Net Carbs 2g; Fat 9g; Protein 51g

Tender Pork Chops with Basil & Beet Greens

Ingredients for 4 servings

2 cups chopped beetroot greens

2 tbsp balsamic vinegar

2 tsp freshly pureed garlic

2 tbsp freshly chopped basil

4 thyme sprigs

1 tbsp olive oil

4 pork chops

2 tbsp butter

Directions and Total Time: approx. 30 minutes

Preheat the oven to 400 F. Add garlic, salt, pepper, vinegar and basil to a saucepan. Cook on low heat until the mixture becomes syrupy. Take a pan and heat olive oil in it and sear the pork. Brush the thyme, vinegar glaze over the pork and bake for 10 minutes. Melt the butter in another pan and saute the beetroot greens. Serve the pork with beetroot greens.

Per serving: Cal 391; Net Carbs 0.8g; Fat 16g; Protein 40g

Ground Pork & Scrambled Eggs with Cabbage

Ingredients for 4 servings

2 tbsp sesame oil

2 large eggs

2 tbsp minced garlic

½ tsp ginger puree

1 medium white onion, diced

1 lb ground pork

1 habanero pepper, chopped

1 green cabbage, shredded

5 scallions, chopped

3 tbsp coconut aminos

1 tbsp white vinegar

2 tbsp sesame seeds

Directions and Total Time: approx. 30 minutes

Heat 1 tsp sesame oil in a pan and scramble the eggs until set and set aside. Heat 1 tsp sesame oil in the same pan and saute ginger, garlic and onion until soft. Add ground pork and habanero pepper and season with salt and pepper. Cook for 10 minutes and mix in the aminos, cabbage, scallions and vinegar. Stir in the egg. Serve garnished with sesame seeds and some low carb tortillas.

Per serving: Cal 295; Net Carbs 3.6g; Fat 16g; Protein 29g

Sweet Pork Chops with Brie Cheese

Ingredients for 4 servings

3 tbsp olive oil

2 large red onions, sliced

2 tbsp balsamic vinegar

1 tsp maple (sugar-free) syrup

Salt and black pepper to taste

4 pork chops

4 slices brie cheese

2 tbsp chopped mint leaves

Directions and Total Time: approx. 45 minutes

Heat 1 tbsp of olive oil in a pan. Reduce the temperature and add the onions. Add vinegar, maple syrup and salt. Cook, stirring frequently to avoid burning, until the onions caramelize and set aside. In the same pan, heat the olive oil and add the pork, salt and pepper and cook for 10 minutes. Place a slice of brie on each meat. Top with caramelized onions; Let the cheese melt for 2 minutes. Spoon meat with toppings onto plates and garnish with mint.

Per serving: Cal 457; Net Carbs 3.1g; Fat 25g; Protein 46g

Sesame Pork Meatballs

Ingredients for 4 servings

1 lb ground pork

2 scallions, chopped

1 zucchini, grated

4 garlic cloves, minced

1 tsp freshly pureed ginger

1 tsp red chili flakes

2 tbsp tamari sauce

2 tbsp sesame oil

3 tbsp coconut oil, for frying

Directions and Total Time: approx. 30 minutes

Take a bowl and combine the pork, zucchini, ginger, chili flakes, garlic, tamari sauce, scallions and sesame oil. With hands, form 1-inch oval shape and place on plate. Take a pan, heat coconut oil on medium heat and brown the balls for 10 minutes. Serve with creamy spinach puree.

Per serving: Cal 296; Net Carbs 1.5g; Fat 22g; Protein 24g

Hot Pork Stir-Fry with Walnuts

Ingredients for 4 servings

1 ½ lb pork tenderloin, cut into strips

2 tbsp coconut oil

Salt and black pepper to taste

1 green bell pepper, diced

1 small red onion, diced

1/3 cup walnuts

1 tbsp freshly grated ginger

3 garlic cloves, minced

1 tsp sesame oil

1 habanero pepper, minced

2 tbsp tamari sauce

Directions and Total Time: approx. 30 minutes

Take a pan, heat coconut oil in it, add pork, salt and pepper and cook for 10 minutes. Shift to one side of the wok and add the onion, walnuts, ginger, bell pepper, garlic, sesame oil, and habanero pepper. Sauté for 5 minutes until onion softens. Season with tamari sauce. Fry until well combined and serve with cauliflower rice.

Per serving: Cal 325; Net Carbs 2.8g; Fat 16g; Protein 38g

Lemony Greek Pork Tenderloin

Ingredients for 4 servings

¼ cup olive oil

2 lemon, juiced

2 tbsp Greek seasoning

2 tbsp red wine vinegar

1 ½ lb pork tenderloin

2 tbsp lard

Directions and Total Time: approx. 2 hours

Preheat the oven to 425 F. Take a bowl and combine olive oil, Greek seasoning, olive oil, vinegar, salt and pepper. Slice the pork and brush the marinade all over. Cover with plastic and refrigerate. Melt the lard in a pan. Place in a greased baking dish, brush with any marinade and bake for 50 minutes. Serve.

Per serving: Cal 383; Net Carbs 2.5g; Fat 24g; Protein 36g

Flavorful Chipotle-Coffee Pork Chops

Ingredients for 4 servings

1 tbsp finely ground coffee

½ tsp chipotle powder

½ tsp garlic powder

½ tsp cinnamon powder

½ tsp cumin powder

1 ½ tsp swerve brown sugar

4 bone-in pork chops

2 tbsp lard

Directions and Total Time: approx. 20 minutes

Take a bowl and mix garlic, cinnamon, coffee, chipotle, cumin, salt, pepper and swerve in it. Season the pork. Cover with plastic wrap and refrigerate overnight. Preheat the oven to 350 F. Melt the lard in a pan and sear the pork for 5 minutes. Transfer the pan to the oven and bake for 10 minutes. Remove to a cutting board, let cool, slice and serve with buttered snap peas.

Per serving: Cal 291; Net Carbs 0.5g; Fat 13g; Protein 39g

Pork Belly with Creamy Coconut Kale

Ingredients for 4 servings

2 lb pork belly, chopped

Salt and black pepper to taste

1 tbsp coconut oil

1 white onion, chopped

6 cloves garlic, minced

¼ cup ginger thinly sliced

4 long red chilies, halved

1 cup coconut milk

1 cup coconut cream

2 cups chopped kale

Directions and Total Time: approx. 40 minutes

Sprinkle the pork belly with salt and pepper and refrigerate for 30 minutes. Take a pot, add 2 cups of water, add pork and boil for 15 minutes. Drain and transfer to a skillet. Fry for 15 minutes. Remove with a spoon to a plate and discard the fat. Heat coconut oil in the same pan and fry garlic, ginger, onion and chillies in it. Add coconut milk and coconut cream and cook. Stir the pork and cook for 2 minutes before serving.

Per serving: Cal 608; Net Carbs 6.7g; Fat 36g; Protein 57g

Pork Medallions with & Morels

Ingredients for 4 servings4

1 ½ lb pork tenderloin, cut into 8 medallions

2 tbsp olive oil

16 fresh morels, rinsed

4 large green onions, chopped

½ cup red wine

¾ cup beef broth

2 tbsp unsalted butter

Directions and Total Time: approx. 25 minutes

Take a pot and heat olive oil in it. Add the pork, sprinkle with salt and pepper and cook for 5 minutes until browned and set aside. Add the green onions and morels and cook for 2 minutes until softened. Mix in mutton broth and red wine. Place the pork in the sauce to simmer. Adjust taste by swirling in butter and serve hot with creamy mashed turnips.

Per serving: Cal 328; Net Carbs 1.2g; Fat 15g; Protein 39g

Mozzarella Baked Pork

Ingredients for 4 servings

4 boneless pork chops

Salt and black pepper to taste

1 cup golden flaxseed meal

1 large egg, beaten

1 cup tomato sauce

1 cup shredded mozzarella

Directions and Total Time: approx. 30 minutes

Preheat the oven to 400 F and grease a baking sheet. Sprinkle the pork with salt and pepper. And take flaxseed meal in a plate. Coat the meat in the egg, then in flaxseed, and place on the baking sheet. Pour tomato sauce over it and sprinkle mozzarella. Bake until cheese melts. Serve hot with salad.

Per serving: Cal 592; Net Carbs 2.7g; Fat 25g; Protein 62g

Juicy Pork Chops with Parmesan

Ingredients for 4 servings

1 lb pork tenderloin, cut into ½-inch medallions

2 cups fresh raspberries

¼ cup water

1 tsp chicken bouillon granules

½ cup almond flour

2 large eggs, lightly beaten

2/3 cup grated Parmesan

Salt and black pepper to taste

6 tbsp butter, divided

1 tsp minced garlic

Sliced fresh raspberries

Directions and Total Time: approx. 30 minutes

Take a blender and add water, chicken granules and raspberries. Process until soft and set aside. Take two more bowls and add parmesan cheese in one and almond flour in the other. Sprinkle salt and pepper over it. Coat first in flour, then in eggs, then in cheese. Take a pan, melt 2 tablespoons of butter in it, add the pork and fry till the meat is cooked inside. Remove to a plate and cover to keep warm. Melt the remaining butter in the same pan and fry the garlic. Stir in the raspberry mixture and cook for 5 minutes. Remove the pork to a dish, spoon the sauce over the top and serve with the spinach.

Per serving: Cal 488; Net Carbs 6.1g; Fat 23g; Protein 34g

Mushroom Pork Meatballs with Parsnips

Ingredients for 4 servings

1 cup cremini mushrooms, chopped

1 ½ lb ground pork

2 garlic cloves, minced

2 small red onions, chopped

1 tsp dried basil

Salt and black pepper to taste

1 cup grated Parmesan

½ almond milk

2 tbsp olive oil

2 cups tomato sauce

6 fresh basil leaves to garnish

1 lb parsnips, chopped

1 cup water

2 tbsp butter

½ cup coconut cream

Directions and Total Time: approx. 60 minutes

Preheat the oven to 350 F. and line a baking tray with parchment paper. Take a bowl and add half the garlic, pork, basil, half the onion, mushrooms, salt and pepper and mix until evenly combined. Mold bite-size balls out of the mixture. Dip each ball first in milk and then in cheese then place on a tray and bake for 25 minutes.

Take a saucepan, heat olive oil in it and saute the remaining garlic and onion. Add tomato sauce and cook for 20 minutes. Add the meatballs and simmer for 10 minutes. Take a pot, add 1 cup of water, parsnips and salt and boil for 10 minutes. Take it in a bowl, add salt, butter, pepper, mash it into a puree using a mash. Stir in Parmesan and coconut cream until combined. Spoon mashed parsnips into bowls, top with meatballs and sauce and garnish with basil leaves.

Per serving: Cal 642; Net Carbs 21.1g; Fat 32g; Protein 50g

Smoked Paprika-Coconut Tenderloin

Ingredients for 4 servings

1 lb pork tenderloin, cubed

4 tsp smoked paprika

Salt and black pepper to taste

1 tsp almond flour

1 tbsp butter

3/4 cup coconut cream

Directions and Total Time: approx. 30 minutes

Pat the pork dry and sprinkle with salt, pepper, almond flour and paprika. Take a pan, melt the butter in it and fry the pork for 7 minutes. Stir in the cream and let it boil. Cook the sauce for 5 minutes. Serve over a bed of coulis rice.

Per serving: Cal 310; Net Carbs 2.5g; Fat 21g; Protein 26g

Mushroom & Pork Casserole

Ingredients for 4 servings

1 cup portobello mushrooms, chopped

1 cup ricotta, crumbled

1 cup Italian cheese blend

4 carrots, thinly sliced

Salt and black pepper to taste

1 clove garlic, minced

1 ¼ pounds ground pork

4 green onions, chopped

15 oz canned tomatoes

4 tbsp pork rinds, crushed

¼ cup chopped parsley

3 tbsp olive oil

⅓ cup water

Directions and Total Time: approx. 38 minutes

Take a bowl and mix the ricotta cheese, eggs and Italian cheese mixture in it and keep aside. Take a kadai, heat olive oil in it and cook the pork for 5 minutes. Add half the green onion, mushrooms, garlic and 2 tablespoons of the pork and cook for 5 minutes. Mix tomatoes with water and cook for 5 minutes. Sprinkle a baking dish with 2 tbsp of pork rinds, top with half of the carrots and a season of salt, 2/3 of the pork mixture, and the cheese mixture. Repeat the layering process a second time to exhaust the ingredients. Cover the baking dish with foil and bake for 30 minutes at 370 F. Remove the foil and brown the top of the casserole with the broiler side of the oven for 5 minutes.

Per serving: Cal 672; Net Carbs 7.9g; Fat 56g; Protein 34.8g

Tangy Lemon Pork Steaks with Mushrooms

Ingredients for 4 servings

8 oz white button mushrooms, chopped

4 large, bone-in pork steaks

2 tsp lemon pepper seasoning

3 tbsp olive oil

3 tbsp butter

1 cup beef stock

6 garlic cloves, minced

2 tbsp chopped parsley

1 lemon, thinly sliced

Directions and Total Time: approx. 30 minutes

Pat the pork dry and season with salt and lemon pepper. Take a pan, heat 2 tablespoons of olive oil and butter on medium heat and cook the meat for 10 minutes and set aside. Add the remaining oil and butter to the pan, add half the stock, mushrooms and garlic to the bottom of the pan and cook for 5 minutes. Return the pork and add the lemon wedges. Garnish the eggs and serve with steamed green beans.

Per serving: Cal 505; Net Carbs 3.2g; Fat 32g; Protein 46g

Celery Braised Pork Shanks in Wine Sauce

Ingredients for 4 servings

3 tbsp olive oil

3 lb pork shanks

3 celery stalks, chopped

5 garlic cloves, minced

1 ½ cups crushed tomatoes

½ cup red wine

¼ tsp red chili flakes

¼ cup chopped parsley

Directions and Total Time: approx. 2 hours 30 minutes

Preheat oven to 300 F. Heat the pork in olive oil in a dutch oven for 5 minutes and set aside. Add garlic and celery and saute for 5 minutes. Return the pork. Top with tomatoes, red wine and chili flakes. Cover the pot and put it in the oven. Cook for 2 hours, turning the meat every 30 minutes. During the last 15 minutes, open the lid and raise the temperature to 450 F. Remove from the pot, stir in the parsley and serve the meat with the sauce on a bed of creamed mashed cauliflower.

Per serving: Cal 520; Net Carbs 1.4g; Fat 20g; Protein 75g

Tuscan Pork Tenderloin with Cauli Rice

Ingredients for 4 servings

1 cup loosely packed fresh baby spinach

2 tbsp olive oil

1 ½ lb pork tenderloin, cubed

Salt and black pepper to taste

½ tsp cumin powder

2 cups cauliflower rice

½ cup water

1 cup grape tomatoes, halved

3/4 cup crumbled feta cheese

Directions and Total Time: approx. 30 minutes

Take a pan and heat olive oil on medium heat. Add pork, salt, pepper and cumin and cook for 5 minutes. Stir the cauli rice and add to the water. Cook until the cauliflower is soft. Mix spinach and add tomatoes. Spoon the dish into bowls, sprinkle with feta cheese and serve with hot sauce.

Per serving: Cal 377; Net Carbs 1.9g; Fat 17g; Protein 43g

Indian Pork Masala

Ingredients for 4 servings

1 ½ lb pork shoulder, cut into bite-size pieces

2 tbsp ghee

1 tbsp freshly grated ginger

2 tbsp freshly pureed garlic

6 medium red onions, sliced

1 cup crushed tomatoes

2 tbsp Greek yogurt

½ tsp chili powder

2 tbsp garam masala

1 bunch cilantro, chopped

2 green chilies, sliced

Directions and Total Time: approx. 30 minutes

Take a pot, boil water in it and blanch the meat for 5 minutes and keep it aside. Take a pan, melt ghee in it and saute onions, garlic and ginger for 5 minutes until caramelized. Mix curd, pork and tomatoes. Sprinkle salt, pepper, chilli and masala on it. Cook for another 10 minutes. Add coriander and green chillies and serve with masala kouli rice.

Per serving: Cal 302; Net Carbs 2.2g; Fat 16g; Protein 33g

Cheesy Sausages in Creamy Onion Sauce

Ingredients for 4 servings

2 tsp almond flour

1 (16 oz) pork sausages

6 tbsp golden flaxseed meal

1 egg, beaten

1 tbsp olive oil

8 oz cream cheese, softened

3 tbsp freshly chopped chives

3 tsp freshly pureed onion

3 tbsp chicken broth

2 tbsp almond milk

Directions and Total Time: approx. 30 minutes

Take a plate, mix flour with salt and pepper and add flaxseed meal to the plate. Prick the sausage with a fork, roll in flour, egg and then flaxseed meal. Heat olive oil in a pan and fry the sausages for 15 minutes. Remove to a plate and cover to keep warm. Take a saucepan and combine onion, cream cheese, stock and milk in it. Cook on medium heat for 5 minutes. Plate the sausages and spoon the sauce on top. Serve immediately with steamed broccoli.

Per serving: Cal 461; Net Carbs 0.5g; Fat 32g; Protein 34g

Savory Jalapeño Pork Meatballs

Ingredients for 4 servings

3 green onions, chopped

1 tbsp garlic powder

1 pound ground pork

1 jalapeño pepper, chopped

1 tsp dried oregano

2 tsp parsley

½ tsp Italian seasoning

2 tsp cumin

Salt and black pepper to taste

3 tbsp butter melted + 2 tbsp

4 ounces cream cheese

1 tsp turmeric

¼ tsp xylitol

½ tsp baking powder

1 ½ cups flax meal

½ cup almond flour

Directions and Total Time: approx. 45 minutes

Preheat the oven to 350 F. Add 1/2 cup water, jalapeno pepper, green onions, garlic powder to a food processor and blend well. Heat 2 tsp of butter in a pan and cook the ground pork for 5 minutes. Stir in the onion mixture and cook for 2 minutes. Add the cumin, cumin, cloves, oregano, 1/2 tsp turmeric, Italian seasoning and pepper and cook for 2 minutes. Take a bowl and combine it with almond flour, remaining turmeric, xylitol, baking powder and flax meal. Form balls of this mixture and set them on parchment paper and roll each one into a circle. Split the pork mixture on one-half of the dough circles, cover with the other half, seal edges, and lay on a lined sheet. Bake for 30 minutes.

Per serving: Cal 598; Net Carbs 5.3g; Fat 45.8g; Protein 35g

Greek-Style Pork Packets with Halloumi

Ingredients for 4 servings

1 lb turnips, cubed

½ cup salsa verde

2 tsp chili powder

1 tsp cumin powder

4 boneless pork chops

Salt and black pepper to taste

3 tbsp olive oil

4 slices halloumi cheese, cubed

Directions and Total Time: approx. 30 minutes

Preheat the oven to 400 F. Cut four 18 x 12 inch sheets of aluminum foil. Grease the sheet with cooking spray. Take a bowl and combine chilies, salsa verde, turnips and cumin. Sprinkle salt and pepper over it. Place a pork chop on each foil sheet, place the turnip mixture on top of the meat, drizzle with olive oil then top with the halloumi cheese. Wrap in foil and place on grill rack and cook for 10 minutes. Flip the foil pack over and cook for another 10 minutes and remove the pack on a plate and serve.

Per serving: Cal 501; Net Carbs 2.1g; Fat 27g; Protein 52g

Hot Pork Chops with Satay Sauce

Ingredients for 4 servings

2 lb boneless pork loin chops, cut into 2-inch pieces

Salt and black pepper to taste

1 medium white onion, sliced

1/3 cup peanut butter

¼ cup tamari sauce

½ tsp garlic powder

½ tsp onion powder

½ tsp hot sauce

1 cup chicken broth, divided

3 tbsp xanthan gum

1 tbsp chopped peanuts

Directions and Total Time: approx. 80 minutes

Take a bowl, add the pork, sprinkle with salt and pepper and add the onion. Take a bowl and combine garlic, peanut butter, tamari sauce and onion powder, hot sauce, two thirds of chicken broth. Pour the mixture over the meat and bring to a boil over high heat. Reduce heat and let simmer for 1 hour. Take a bowl and mix the remaining mutton broth and xantham gum in it, stir the mixture into the mutton and boil for 2 minutes. Garnish on a plate and serve.

Per serving: Cal 455; Net Carbs 6.7g; Fat 17g; Protein 61g

Turnip Pork Pie

Ingredients for 8 servings

1 cup turnip mash

2 pounds ground pork

½ cup water

1 onion, chopped

1 tbsp sage

2 tbsp butter

Crust:

2 oz butter

1 egg

2 oz cheddar, shredded

2 cups almond flour

¼ tsp xanthan gum

A pinch of salt

Directions and Total Time: approx. 50 minutes

Cook bacon in skillet until crisp. Place on a paper towel lined plate. Heat 1 tsp of olive oil in a pan and fry the mushrooms in it. Sprinkle salt and pepper on it and cook for 5 minutes. Heat the remaining oil and fry the pork in it for 10 minutes. Let cool. and add in turnip mash and sage. Roll out the pie crusts and place one at the bottom of a greased pie pan. Spread filling over the crust and top with the other coat. Bake in the oven for 35 minutes at 350 F. Serve.

Per serving: Cal 477; Net Carbs 1.7g; Fat 36.1g; Protein 33g

Sweet Pork Chops with Hoisin Sauce

Ingredients for 4 servings

4 oz hoisin sauce, sugar-free

1 ¼ pounds pork chops

Salt and black pepper to taste

1 tbsp xylitol

½ tsp ginger powder

2 tsp smoked paprika

Directions and Total Time: approx. 2 hours 20 minutes

Take a bowl and mix xylitol, ginger, pepper and paprika in it. Spread the mixture over the pork. Cover with a plastic lid and refrigerate for 2 hours. Heat the grill and grill the meat on each side. Reduce heat and brush with hoisin sauce, cover and grill for 7 minutes. Brush with hoisin sauce and cook for another 5 minutes.

Per serving: Cal 352; Net Carbs 2.5g; Fat 22.9g; Protein 37g

Basil Pork Meatballs in Tomato Sauce

Ingredients for 6 servings

1 pound ground pork

2 green onions, chopped

1 tbsp olive oil

1 cup pork rinds, crushed

3 cloves garlic, minced

½ cup buttermilk

2 eggs, beaten

1 cup asiago cheese, shredded

Salt and black pepper to taste

1 can (29-ounce) tomato sauce

1 cup pecorino cheese, grated

Chopped basil to garnish

Directions and Total Time: approx. 45 minutes

Preheat the oven to 370 F. Take a bowl and mix the ground pork, buttermilk, garlic, Asiago cheese, salt, pepper, egg and pork until combined. Form the pork mixture into balls and place in a greased baking pan. Bake for 25 minutes and remove. Sprinkle with pecorino cheese and add to tomato sauce. Cover the pan with foil and place in the oven for 10 minutes. Remove the foil and cook for another 7 minutes. Garnish with basil and serve.

Per serving: Cal 623; Net Carbs 4.6g; Fat 51.8g; Protein 53g

Canadian Pork Pie

Ingredients for 8 servings

1 cup cooked and mashed cauliflower

1 egg

¼ cup butter

2 cups almond flour

¼ tsp xanthan gum

¼ cup shredded mozzarella

2 pounds ground pork

⅓ cup pureed onion

¾ tsp allspice

1 tbsp ground sage

2 tbsp butter

Directions and Total Time: approx. 1 hour 40 minutes

Preheat the oven to 350 F. Take a bowl and whisk butter, almond flour, egg, mozzarella cheese, salt in it. Make 2 balls of the mixture and refrigerate for 10 minutes. Melt the butter in a pan and cook the salt, onion, ground pork and spices for 5 minutes. Take out in a bowl and mix with the flower and sage. Scoop out the pie balls and place in the bottom of a greased pie pan. Spread the pork mixture over the crust. Bake for 50 minutes and serve.

Per serving: Cal 485; Net Carbs 4g; Fat 41g; Protein 29g

Quick Pork Lo Mein

Ingredients for 4 servings

4 boneless pork chops, cut into ¼-inch strips

1 cup green beans, halved

1 cup shredded mozzarella

1 egg yolk

1-inch ginger knob, grated

3 tbsp sesame oil

Salt and black pepper to taste

1 red bell pepper, sliced

1 yellow bell pepper, sliced

1 garlic clove, minced

4 green onions, chopped

1 tsp toasted sesame seeds

3 tbsp coconut aminos

2 tsp sugar-free maple syrup

1 tsp fresh ginger paste

Directions and Total Time: approx. 25 min + chilling time

Heat mozzarella cheese in microwave for 2 minutes and let it cool for 2 minutes. Mix the egg yolks until combined. Place the parchment paper on top of the cheese mixture and cover with another parchment paper. Flatten the dough to 1/8 inch thickness. Remove the parchment paper and cut the dough into thin spaghetti strands.

Place in a bowl and refrigerate overnight. Boil 2 cups of water in a saucepan and add the pasta. Cook and keep aside. Heat sesame oil in a pan. Season the pork on both sides with salt and pepper. Remove in a plate. In the same kadai, mix farsabi, bell pepper and cook for 5 minutes. Stir in the green onions, garlic and ginger and cook for 1 minute. Add the pork and pasta to the pan. Take a bowl and add remaining sesame oil, coconut aminos, maple syrup and ginger paste in it. Serve.

Per serving: Cal 338; Fats 12g; Net Carbs 4.6g; Protein 43g

Tasty Sambal Pork Noodles

Ingredients for 4 servings

2 (8 oz) packs Miracle noodles, garlic, and herb

1 tbsp olive oil

1 lb ground pork

4 garlic cloves, minced

1-inch ginger, grated

1 tsp liquid stevia

1 tbsp tomato paste

2 fresh basil leaves, chopped

2 tbsp sambal oelek

2 tbsp plain vinegar

2 tbsp coconut aminos

Salt to taste

1 tbsp unsalted butter

Directions and Total Time: approx. 60 minutes

Take a bowl, take 2 cups of water, add miracle noodles to it, filter it and wash it well. Add back to boiling water and cook for 4 minutes. In a dry pan, fry the shirataki noodles for 2 minutes until dry. Add salt and keep aside. Heat olive oil in a pot and cook for 5 minutes. Add tomato paste and mix with 1 cup water, vinegar, aminos and salt. Reduce the heat and cook for 35 minutes. Add butter and mix well with shirataki sauce. Serve.

Per serving: Cal 505; Fats 30g; Net Carbs 8.2g; Protein 34g

Baked Tenderloin with Lime Chimichurri

Ingredients for 4 servings

1 lime, juiced

¼ cup chopped mint leaves

¼ cup rosemary, chopped

2 cloves garlic, minced

¼ cup olive oil

4 lb pork tenderloin

Salt and black pepper to taste

Olive oil for rubbing

Directions and Total Time: approx. 1 hour 10 minutes

Take a bowl and mix together lemon juice, mint, rosemary, olive oil and salt. Keep aside. Preheat a charcoal grill to 450 F. Brush the pork with olive oil and sprinkle with salt and pepper. Keep the heat and cook the meat for 5 minutes. Close the lid and cook on one side for 20 minutes. Flip open and grill for 20 minutes. Serve.

Per serving: Cal 388, Net Carbs 2.1g, Fat 18g, Protein 28g

Green Bean Creamy Pork with Fettuccine

Ingredients for 4 servings

4 pork loin medallions, cut into thin strips

1 cup shredded mozzarella

1 cup shaved Parmesan cheese

1 egg yolk

1 tbsp olive oil

Salt and black pepper to taste

½ cup green beans, chopped

1 lemon, zested and juiced

¼ cup chicken broth

1 cup crème fraiche

6 basil leaves, chopped

Directions and Total Time: approx. 40 min + chilling time

Put the mozzarella cheese in the microwave for 2 minutes and heat it up. Mix in the egg yolks until well combined. Place cheese mixture on parchment paper and cover with another parchment paper. Flatten the dough to 1/8 inch thickness. Remove the parchment paper and cut the dough into thick fettuccine strands. Place in a bowl and refrigerate overnight.

Boil 2 cups of water in a saucepan and add the fettuccine. Cook for 2 minutes and remove. Keep aside. Take a pan and heat olive oil in it. Season the pork with pepper and salt and cook for 10 minutes. Mix in the green beans and cook for another 5 minutes. Stir in chicken broth and lemon juice. Cook for another 6-7 minutes. Add crème fraiche, fettuccine, and basil and cook for 1 minute. Top with Parmesan cheese. Serve.

Per serving: Cal 586; Fats 32.3g; Net Carbs 9g; Protein 59g

Cauliflower Pork Goulash

Ingredients for 4 servings

2 tbsp butter

1 cup mushrooms, sliced

1 ½ pounds ground pork

Salt and black pepper, to taste

2 cups cauliflower florets

1 onion, chopped

14 ounces canned tomatoes

1 garlic clove, minced

1 tbsp smoked paprika

2 tbsp parsley, chopped

1 tbsp tomato puree

1 ½ cups water

Directions and Total Time: approx. 30 minutes

Take a pan and melt butter in it on medium flame. Stir in the pork and cook for 5 minutes. Put in the garlic, onion and mushrooms and cook for 5 minutes. Stir in the tomato paste, water, paprika, tomatoes and flour. Boil and cook for 20 minutes. Add eggs, pepper and salt and serve.

Per serving: Cal 533; Net Carbs 7g; Fat 41.8g; Protein 35.5g

Basil Prosciutto Pizza

Ingredients for 4 servings

4 prosciutto slices, cut into thirds

2 cups grated mozzarella cheese

2 tbsp cream cheese, softened

½ cup almond flour

1 egg, beaten

⅓ cup tomato sauce

⅓ cup sliced mozzarella

6 fresh basil leaves, to serve

Directions and Total Time: approx. 45 minutes

Preheat oven to 390 F. Line a pizza pan with parchment paper. Microwave the mozzarella cheese and cream cheese for 1 minute. Mix in almond meal and egg. Spread the mixture on a pizza pan and bake for 20 minutes. Keep aside. Spread the tomato sauce over the crust. Add the mozzarella slices over the sauce and bake for 15 minutes. Top with tulsi and curry leaves and serve in slices.

Per serving: Cal 160; Net Carbs 0.5g; Fats 6.2g; Protein 22g

Bell Pepper Noodles with Pork Avocado

Ingredients for 4 servings

2 lb red and yellow bell peppers, spiralized

2 tbsp butter

1 lb ground pork

Salt and black pepper to taste

1 tsp garlic powder

2 avocados, pitted, mashed

2 tbsp chopped pecans

Directions and Total Time: approx. 15 minutes

Take a pan, melt the butter in it and cook the pork for 5 minutes. Sprinkle salt and pepper over it. Add garlic powder, bell pepper and stir. Add chillies and cook for 2 minutes. Mix in the mashed avocado. Serve.

Per serving: Cal 704; Fats 49g; Net Carbs 9.3g; Protein 35g

Caribbean Jerk Pork

Ingredients for 4 servings

1 ½ pounds pork roast

1 tbsp olive oil

¼ cup jerk seasoning

2 tbsp soy sauce, sugar-free

½ cup vegetable stock

Directions and Total Time: approx. 4 hours 20 minutes

Preheat oven to 350 F and drizzle olive oil and jerk seasoning over pork. Take a pan, heat olive oil on medium heat and fry the meat for 5 minutes. Place the pork in a baking dish and add the vegetable stock and soy sauce. Cover with aluminum foil and bake for 50 minutes. Flip halfway through then remove the foil and cook completely. Serve.

Per serving: Cal 407; Net Carbs 5.6g; Fat 20g; Protein 46g

Parmesan Pork with Green Pasta

Ingredients for 4 servings

4 boneless pork chops

Salt and black pepper to taste

½ cup basil pesto

1 cup grated Parmesan cheese

1 tbsp butter

4 large turnips, spiralized

Directions and Total Time: approx. 1 hour 30 minutes

Preheat the oven to 350 F. Season the pork with salt and pepper. and place on a greased baking dish. Spread the pesto over the pork and bake for 50 minutes. Take out the baking sheet. Divide the Parmesan cheese in half and pour over the pork. Cook for another 5 minutes and keep aside. Melt the butter in a pan and fry the turnips for 5 minutes. Serve the pork on plates.

Per serving: Cal 532; Fats 28g; Net Carbs 4.9g; Protein 54g

Grilled BBQ Pork Chops

Ingredients for 4 servings

4 pork loin chops, boneless

½ cup sugar-free BBQ sauce

1 tbsp erythritol

½ tsp ginger powder

½ tsp garlic powder

2 tsp smoked paprika

Directions and Total Time: approx. 1 hour 50 minutes

Take a bowl and mix black pepper, ginger powder, erythritol, smoked paprika and garlic powder in it. and sear all sides of the pork chops. Cover the pork chops with plastic wrap in the refrigerator for 1 hour. Heat the grill and place the meat on it and cook it on all sides. Reduce heat to low and brush with BBQ sauce. Serve.

Per serving: Cal 363, Net Carbs 0g, Fat 26.6g, Protein 34.1g

Pecorino Romano Kohlrabi with Sausage

Ingredients for 4 servings

1 cup grated Pecorino Romano cheese

2 tbsp olive oil

1 cup sliced pork sausage

4 bacon slices, chopped

4 large kohlrabi, spiralized

6 garlic cloves, minced

1 cup cherry tomatoes, halved

7 fresh basil leaves

1 tbsp pine nuts for topping

Directions and Total Time: approx. 15 minutes

Take a pan and heat olive oil in it. Cook for 5 minutes until sausage and bacon are browned. Remove in a plate. Stir in the garlic and kohlrabi and cook for 5 minutes until softened. Add salt, pepper, cherry tomatoes and cook for 2 minutes. Mix in the sausage, bacon, basil and Pecorino Romano cheese. Garnish with pine nuts and serve hot.

Per serving: Cal 229; Fats 20.2g; Net Carbs 2.4g; Protein 8g

Chorizo Smoky Pizza

Ingredients for 4 servings

2 cups shredded mozzarella

1 cup sliced smoked mozzarella

2 tbsp cream cheese, softened

¾ cup almond flour

2 tbsp almond meal

1 tbsp olive oil

1 cups sliced chorizo

¼ cup marinara sauce

1 jalapeño pepper, sliced

¼ red onion, thinly sliced

Directions and Total Time: approx. 45 minutes

Preheat the oven to 390 F. Line a pizza pan with parchment paper. Microwave the cream cheese and mozzarella cheese for 25 seconds. Remove the almond flour and mix it with the almond meal. Spread the mixture on the pizza pan and bake for 10 minutes. Heat olive oil and cook for 5 minutes. Spread the marinara sauce over the crust and add the chorizo, jalapeño peppers, onion and smoked mozzarella cheese. Bake for 15 minutes. Remove, slice and serve.

Per serving: Cal 302; Net Carbs 1.4g; Fats 17g; Protein 31g

Monterey Jack & Sausage-Pepper Pizza

Ingredients for 4 servings

1 ½ lb Italian pork sausages, crumbled

½ cup grated Monterey Jack cheese

1 cup chopped bell peppers

4 cups grated mozzarella

¼ cup grated Parmesan

2 tbsp cream cheese, softened

¼ cup coconut flour

1 cup almond flour

2 eggs

1 tbsp olive oil

1 onion, thinly sliced

2 garlic cloves, minced

1 cup baby spinach

½ cup sugar-free pizza sauce

Directions and Total Time: approx. 45 minutes

Preheat the oven to 390 F and line a pizza pan with parchment paper. Microwave 2 tablespoons of cream cheese and mozzarella cheese for 1 minute. Mix the sausage, parmesan cheese, egg, almond flour and coconut flour. Spread the mixture on a pizza pan and bake for 15 minutes and set aside. Take a pan, heat olive oil and saute garlic, bell pepper and onion in it. Stir in spinach and allow wilting for 3 minutes. Spread the pizza sauce on the crust and top with the bell pepper mixture. Scatter mozzarella and Monterey Jack cheeses on top. Bake for 5 minutes.

Per serving: Cal 460; Net Carbs 3g; Fats 25.6g; Protein 47g

Maple Pork with Spaghetti Squash

Ingredients for 4 servings

3 lb spaghetti squashes, halved and deseeded

2 tbsp minced lemongrass

3 tbsp fresh ginger paste

2 tbsp sugar-free maple syrup

2 tbsp coconut aminos

1 tbsp fish sauce

4 boneless pork chops

3 tbsp peanut oil

1 tbsp olive oil

Salt and black pepper to taste

1 lb baby spinach

½ cup coconut milk

¼ cup peanut butter

Directions and Total Time: approx. 1 hour + marinating

Take a bowl and mix maple syrup, 2 teaspoons of ginger paste, lemongrass, aminos and fish sauce in it. Place the pork in the liquid and coat well. Marinate for 50 minutes. Take a pan, heat 2 tablespoons of groundnut oil in it, remove the pork from the marinade and sear for 15 minutes. Remove in a plate and keep covered. Preheat the oven to 380 F. Place spaghetti squash on a baking sheet, brush with olive oil and season with salt and pepper.

Bake for 50 minutes. Remove squash and shred into spaghetti-like strands with two forks. Keep warm. Heat the remaining groundnut oil in the same pan and fry the remaining ginger paste. Add spinach and cook for 2 minutes and keep aside. Take a bowl and whisk the coconut milk with the peanut butter until well combined. Slice the pork and top with the spinach and peanut sauce and serve immediately.

Per serving: Cal 694; Fats 34g; Net Carbs 7.6g; Protein 53g

Spicy Grilled Pork Spareribs

Ingredients for 4 servings

4 tbsp sugar-free BBQ sauce + extra for serving

2 tbsp erythritol

1 tbsp olive oil

3 tsp cayenne powder

1 tsp garlic powder

1 lb pork spareribs

Directions and Total Time: approx. 2 hours

Mix erythritol, salt, pepper, oil, cayenne, and garlic. Brush on the meaty sides of the ribs and wrap in foil. Sit for 30 minutes to marinate. Preheat the oven to 400 F, place the ribs on a baking sheet and cook for 40 minutes. Remove foil, brush with BBQ sauce and cook under broiler until browned on both sides. Slice and serve.

Per serving: Cal 395, Net Carbs 3g, Fat 33g, Protein 21g

Asian-Style Pork and Celeriac Noodles

Ingredients for 4 servings

3 tbsp sugar-free maple syrup

3 tbsp coconut aminos

1 tbsp fresh ginger paste

¼ tsp Chinese five spice

Salt and black pepper to taste

1 lb pork tenderloin, cubed

2 tbsp butter

4 large celeriac, spiralized

1 tbsp sesame oil

24 oz bok choy, chopped

2 green onions, chopped

2 tbsp sesame seeds

Directions and Total Time: approx. 1 hour 20 minutes

Preheat the oven to 400 F and line a baking sheet with foil. Take a bowl and mix coconut aminos, maple syrup, Chinese 5 spice powder, ginger paste, salt and pepper in it. Set aside 4 tablespoons of the mixture for a little topping. Mix the pork with the remaining marinade and marinate for 30 minutes. Take a pan, melt the butter and saute the celery. Keep aside. Remove the pork from the marinade to a baking sheet and bake for 50 minutes. Heat sesame oil in a wok and saute the bok choy and celeriac pasta for 2 minutes. Transfer to a serving bowl and top with pork. Garnish with green onions and sesame seeds. Drizzle with reserved marinade and serve.

Per serving: Cal 409; Fats 17.8g; Net Carbs 3g; Protein 44g

Pulled Pork Tenderloin with Avocado

Ingredients for 8 servings

4 pounds pork tenderloin

1 tbsp avocado oil

½ cup chicken stock

¼ cup jerk seasoning

6 avocado, sliced

Salt and black pepper to taste

Directions and Total Time: approx. 2 hours

Grease a baking dish and place the pork shoulder in the dish with the seasoning. Add the stock and cover with aluminum foil and cook in the oven at 350 F for 1 hour and 30 minutes. Discard the foil and cook for another 20 minutes. Cut into pieces and serve topped with avocado slices.

Per serving: Cal 567, Net Carbs 4.1g, Fat 42.6g, Protein 42g

Broccoli Tips with Lemon Pork Chops

Ingredients for 6 servings

1 lb fresh broccoli tips, halved

3 tbsp lemon juice

3 cloves garlic, pureed

1 tbsp olive oil

6 pork loin chops

1 tbsp butter

2 tbsp white wine

Directions and Total Time: approx. 30 minutes

Preheat broiler to 400 F. And mix garlic, lemon juice, garlic, salt, pepper and oil in a bowl. Spread the mixture over the pork and place in a baking sheet. and cook until browned on each side. Divide among 6 plates. Melt the butter in a small pan and cook the broccoli tips until tender. Sprinkle with salt, pepper and white wine and cook for 5 minutes. Ladle the broccoli alongside the chops and serve with the hot sauce.

Per serving: Cal 549, Net Carbs 2g, Fat 48g, Protein 26g

Jerk Pork Pot Roast

Ingredients for 8 servings

4-pound pork roast

1 tbsp olive oil

¼ cup Jerk spice blend

½ cup beef stock

Directions and Total Time: approx. 4 hours 20 minutes

Rub the pork with the spice mix and olive oil. Heat a dutch oven to medium heat. Season the meat well on all sides. Reduce the heat and cover the pot and let it cook for 4 hours. Serve.

Per serving: Cal 282; Net Carbs 0g; Fat 24g; Protein 23g

Swiss Pork Patties with Salad

Ingredients for 4 servings

1 lb ground pork

3 tbsp olive oil

2 hearts romaine lettuce, torn

2 firm tomatoes, sliced

¼ red onion, sliced

3 oz Swiss cheese, shredded

Directions and Total Time: approx. 30 minutes

Season pork with salt and pepper, mix, and shape several medium-sized patties. Take a pan, heat 2 tbsp of oil in it and fry the patties on both sides. Drain the oil in a wire rack and once cool, cut into cubes. Mix onion, lettuce, oil, tomatoes, salt and pepper in a bowl. Toss and top with patties. Microwave cheese for 60 seconds, drizzle over salad.

Per serving: Cal 310, Net Carbs 2g, Fat 23g, Protein 22g

Maple Scallion Pork Bites

Ingredients for 4 servings

½ cup + 1 tbsp red wine

1 tbsp + 1/3 cup tamari sauce

1 pork tenderloin, cubed

½ cup sugar-free maple syrup

½ cup sesame seeds

1 tbsp sesame oil

1 tsp freshly pureed garlic

½ tsp freshly grated ginger

1 scallion, finely chopped

Directions and Total Time: approx. 50 minutes

Preheat the oven to 350 F. Combine 1/2 cup red wine with 1 tablespoon tamari sauce in a zipper bag. Add the pork cubes, seal the bag and marinate the meat in the fridge overnight. Remove from fridge. Take sesame seeds and maple syrup in two separate bowls. Roll the pork in the maple syrup and then in the sesame seeds. Place on a greased baking sheet and bake for 40 minutes. In a bowl, mix the tamari sauce, sesame oil, garlic, remaining wine and ginger. Scoop the sauce into a bowl and remove the pork to a plate. Serve with sauce.

Per serving: Cal 352; Net Carbs 6.4g; Fat 18g; Protein 39g

Pork Medallions with Pancetta

Ingredients for 4 servings

1 lb pork loin, cut into medallions

2 onions, chopped

6 pancetta slices, chopped

½ cup vegetable stock

Salt and black pepper, to taste

Directions and Total Time: approx. 55 minutes

Set a pan over a medium heat and cook the pancetta until crisp and remove to a plate. Add onions to it and saute. set aside to the same plate as the pancetta. Add pepper, pork medallions and salt to the pan. Brown on each side and cook on low heat for 5 minutes. Stir in the stock. Stir in the pancetta and onions and cook for 1 minute.

Per serving: Cal 325, Net Carbs 6g, Fat 18g, Protein 36g

Golden Pork Chops with Mushrooms

Ingredients for 6 servings

2 (14-oz) cans Mushroom soup

1 onion, chopped

6 pork chops

½ cup sliced mushrooms

Salt and black pepper to taste

Directions and Total Time: approx. 1 hour 15 minutes

Preheat the oven to 375 F. Season the pork chops with pepper and salt and place in a baking dish. Take a pot and combine onions, soup and mushrooms in it. Pour this mixture over the pork chops and bake for 50 minutes.

Per serving: Cal 403; Net Carbs 8g; Fat 32.6g; Protein 19g

Cumin Pork Chops

Ingredients for 4 servings

4 pork chops

¾ cup cumin powder

1 tsp chili powder

Salt and black pepper to taste

Directions and Total Time: approx. 25 minutes

Take a bowl and combine cumin seeds with chili, black pepper and salt. Place in the porkchops and rub them well. Heat the grill to medium heat and cook the pork for 5 minutes. Serve.

Per serving: Cal 349; Net Carbs 4g; Fat 18.6g; Protein 42g

Crusted Pork Loin

Preparation time: 10 minutes

Cooking time: 1 hour and 10 minutes

Servings: 8

Ingredients:

3 tablespoons mustard

2 tablespoons ghee, melted

1 tablespoon stevia

¼ cup dill, chopped

3 green onions, chopped

1 tablespoon lemon peel, grated

A pinch of salt and black pepper

1 pork loin, boneless

Directions:

Take a bowl and whisk mustard, stevia and mustard together. Take another bowl and mix in fennel, lemon peel and spring onions. Sprinkle pepper and salt over the pork and mix in the mustard. Place the pork in the pan and cook in the oven at 375 F for 1 hour and 10 minutes. Slice and divide into plates and serve with salad.

Nutrition: calories 221, fat 3, fiber 5, carbs 14, protein 20

Glazed Pork Chops

Preparation time: 10 minutes

Cooking time: 12 minutes

Servings: 4

Ingredients:

4 pork chops, bone-in

2 tablespoons stevia

1 tablespoon balsamic vinegar

4 tablespoons ghee, melted

4 ounces baby spinach

Directions:

Heat ghee in a pan on medium heat. Toss with pork chops, vinegar and stevia and add to preheated

broiler. Cook on medium heat on each side. Divide the pork between plates, heat a pan with the glaze over medium heat, add the spinach, cook for about 3 minutes, divide between plates and serve.

Nutrition: calories 321, fat 13, fiber 3, carbs 12, protein 20

Pork Meatballs

Preparation time: 10 minutes

Cooking time: 12 minutes

Servings: 4

Ingredients:

½ cup carrots, grated

¼ cup mint, chopped

3 garlic cloves, minced

1 shallot, chopped

1 lemongrass stalk, chopped

1 pound pork, ground

1 teaspoon hot sauce

1 tablespoon cilantro, chopped

2 tablespoons olive oil

Directions:

Take a bowl and combine the mint, carrot, garlic, lemongrass, peanuts, pork coriander and hot sauce and stir to form medium meatballs. Heat a pan with oil on medium high heat. Add meatballs, cook on each side, remove to plates and serve with salad.

Nutrition: calories 261, fat 13, fiber 7, carbs 13, protein 14

Pork and Asparagus

Preparation time: 10 minutes

Cooking time: 20 minutes

Servings: 4

Ingredients:

4 pork loin chops, boneless

2 tablespoons tarragon, chopped

A pinch of salt and black pepper

1 pound asparagus, trimmed and halved

2 tablespoons olive oil

1 bunch green onions, chopped

½ cup veggie stock

1 tablespoon mustard

Directions:

Heat a pan with oil on medium high heat. Add the pork, season with salt, pepper and tarragon, cook on each side and remove to a bowl. Again heat the same pan on medium heat and add green onions, asparagus and stir fry for 5 minutes. Add the mustard and stock and cook for a further 2 minutes. Return the pork to the pan, cook for a further 5 minutes, remove to plates and serve.

Nutrition: calories 300, fat 9, fiber 2, carbs 14, protein 20

Easy Pulled Pork

Preparation time: 10 minutes

Cooking time: 2 hours and 30 minutes

Servings: 4

Ingredients:

1 pound pork tenderloin, sliced

2 tablespoons chili powder

½ cup tomato paste

2 tablespoons mustard

2 tablespoons olive oil

2 tablespoon balsamic vinegar

A pinch of salt and black pepper

Directions:

Take oil in a pan and grease it. Add the pork tenderloin slices. Add tomato paste, chilli powder, mustard, oil, vinegar, salt and pepper, mix well and cover with a dish. Place in the oven and cook for 2 hours and 30 minutes. Chop the meat and take it out in plates and serve with salad.

Nutrition: calories 264, fat 11, fiber 8, carbs 12, protein 20

Delicious Pork Tenderloin

Preparation time: 10 minutes

Cooking time: 37 minutes

Servings: 6

Ingredients:

2 pounds pork tenderloin

2 lemons, sliced

4 teaspoons olive oil

A pinch of salt and black pepper

2 garlic cloves, minced

2 bunches Swiss chard, chopped

Directions:

Place pork tenderloin on a lined baking sheet, season with salt, pepper, oil, garlic and lemon wedges and cook in oven at 450 F for 30 minutes. Add the Swiss chard, toss and cook in the oven for 5 minutes. Slice the pork and remove to plates and serve.

Nutrition: calories 312, fat 11, fiber 5, carbs 15, protein 18

Slow Cooked Ribs

Preparation time: 10 minutes

Cooking time: 4 hours

Servings: 4

Ingredients:

2 pounds baby back ribs

A pinch of salt and black pepper

1 cup tomato sauce

1 tablespoon balsamic vinegar

2 garlic cloves, minced

1 teaspoon sesame seeds

Directions:

Combine ribs in slow cooker with tomato sauce, vinegar, garlic, salt and pepper. Toss, cover and cook for 4 hours. Divide ribs between plates, sprinkle sesame seeds all over and serve.

Nutrition: calories 294, fat 11, fiber 2, carbs 16, protein 30

Pork Chops and Apricot Sauce

Preparation time: 10 minutes

Cooking time: 15 minutes

Servings: 4

Ingredients:

4 pork chops, bone-in

1 tablespoon olive oil

½ cup veggie stock

¼ cup apricot jam

3 tablespoons mustard

A pinch of salt and black pepper

Directions:

Take a pan and heat oil on medium high temperature. Add the pork chops, cook on each side and divide between plates. Heat the same pan again over medium heat and stir in the jam, mustard, salt, stock and pepper. Cook for 5 minutes and serve drizzled over the pork chops.

Nutrition: calories 321, fat 7, fiber 5, carbs 14, protein 20

Vietnamese Salad

Preparation time: 10 minutes

Cooking time: 10 minutes

Servings: 4

Ingredients:

3 tablespoons coconut aminos

2 tablespoons stevia

2 tablespoons white vinegar

1 tablespoon olive oil

1 pound pork, ground

1 jalapeno, chopped

1 romaine lettuce heart, sliced

¼ cup mint, chopped

3 garlic cloves, minced

Directions:

Take a pan Heat the pan with oil on medium high temperature. Stir in the pork and cook for 5 minutes. Stir in the stevia, coconut aminos, jalapeño, mint, and garlic. Take a bowl and toss the pork, lettuce in it.

Nutrition: calories 342, fat 12, fiber 4, carbs 13, protein 28

Grilled Pork and Mango Salsa

Preparation time: 10 minutes

Cooking time: 6 minutes

Servings: 4

Ingredients:

4 pork loin chops, boneless

2 tablespoons olive oil

1 teaspoon chili powder

A pinch of salt and black pepper

1 mango, peeled and chopped

1 tomato, cubed

1 teaspoon balsamic vinegar

Directions

Heat half the oil in a pan over medium heat and add the pork chops. Add salt, pepper and chili powder. Cook on each side and remove to a plate. Take a bowl and toss together the mango with the vinegar and tomatoes. Serve.

Nutrition: calories 290, fat 12, fiber 4, carbs 14, protein 8

Pork Roast and Cabbage

Preparation time: 10 minutes

Cooking time: 32 minutes

Servings: 4

Ingredients:

2 tablespoons olive oil

1 pork tenderloin

¼ cup tomato sauce

1 red cabbage head, shredded

4 green onions, chopped

2 tablespoons balsamic vinegar

1 jalapeno, chopped

Directions:

Heat half the oil in a pan on medium heat. Cook the pork until browned on each side. Remove to roasting pan and brush with tomato sauce. Bake in the oven at 450 F for 15 minutes. Slice and take out in a plate. Heat a pan on medium heat. Add cabbage, jalapeño, green onions and vinegar. Toss and cook for 10 minutes. Serve with roast pork.

Nutrition: calories 300, fat 12, fiber 9, carbs 18, protein 30

Pork and Apples

Preparation time: 10 minutes

Cooking time: 1 hour and 10 minutes

Servings: 8

Ingredients:

1 pork loin, boneless

1 and ½ teaspoon red pepper, crushed

2 tablespoons olive oil

3 apples, cored and cut into wedges

2 yellow onions, cut into wedges

2 tablespoons ghee, melted

¼ cup apple vinegar

2 teaspoons cinnamon powder

3 star anise

5 garlic slices, chopped

1 tablespoon parsley, chopped

Directions:

Place the pork in a pan. Add the apples, red pepper, oil, onions, ghee, vinegar, star anise, garlic and scallions and toss. Place in oven and cook at 400 F for 1 hour. Divide between plates and serve with apple mix on the side.

Nutrition: calories 321, fat 10, fiber 4, carbs 13, protein 20

Fried Pork Chops

Preparation time: 10 minutes

Cooking time: 10 minutes

Servings: 4

Ingredients:

1 cup olive oil

1 pound pork chops, boneless

A pinch of salt and black pepper

½ cup coconut flour

Directions:

Season the pork with salt and pepper and toss in the coconut batter. Heat oil over medium high heat and add pork chops and cook on each side. Divide between plates and serve with salad.

Nutrition: calories 299, fat 4, fiber 6, carbs 14, protein 18

Pork Chops and Arugula Mix

Preparation time: 10 minutes

Cooking time: 12 minutes

Servings: 4

Ingredients:

4 pork chops, bone-in

A pinch of salt and black pepper

¼ cup capers

3 garlic cloves, minced

1 cup basil, chopped

1 cup parsley, chopped

5 cups baby arugula

1 cup olive oil+ 1 tablespoon

Juice of 1 lemon

Directions:

In a blender, combine the basil, eggs, capers, garlic, lentils, and 1 cup arugula. Spread this over the pork chops. Take a pan and heat 1 cup of oil on medium heat. Cook on each side and divide between plates. Take a bowl, toss together lemon juice and remaining oil and serve.

Nutrition: calories 311, fat 4, fiber 8, carbs 12, protein 7

Meatball Soup

Preparation time: 10 minutes

Cooking time: 10 minutes

Servings: 4

Ingredients:

1 pound pork, ground

3 garlic cloves, minced

2 green onions, chopped

1-inch ginger, grated

1-quart chicken stock

1 cup spinach, torn

A pinch of salt and black pepper

Directions:

Take a bowl and combine garlic, green onions, pork, ginger, salt and pepper. Stir and shape the mixture into meatballs. Add to preheated broiler and cook for 5 minutes. Heat pot with stock over medium-high heat, add meatballs, salt, pepper and spinach, toss, cook for another 5 minutes, ladle into bowls and serve.

Nutrition: calories 300, fat 3, fiber 7, carbs 12, protein 14

Pork Chops and Peperonata

Preparation time: 10 minutes

Cooking time: 10 minutes

Servings: 4

Ingredients:

5 teaspoons olive oil

4 pork loin chops, bone-in

A pinch of salt and black pepper

1 cup red onion, chopped

4 garlic cloves, minced

1 poblano chili, chopped

1 red bell pepper, chopped

1 yellow bell pepper, chopped

3 tablespoons parsley, chopped

2 tablespoons capers

3 tablespoons red vinegar

¼ teaspoon red pepper, crushed

Directions:

Take a pan and heat half oil in it on medium high temperature. Add pork chops to it. Season with salt and pepper and cook for 3 minutes on each side and remove to plates. Heat the same skillet with the remaining oil over medium-high heat and add the onion, garlic, poblano, and bell pepper. Add vinegar, capers, eggs and crushed red pepper and cook for 2 minutes. and serve.

Nutrition: calories 265, fat 11, fiber 4, carbs 14, protein 20

Garam Masala Pork Shoulder

Ingredients for 4 servings

2 tbsp ghee

1 ½ lb pork shoulder, cubed

1 tbsp freshly grated ginger

2 tbsp pureed garlic

6 red onions, sliced

1 cup crushed tomatoes

2 tbsp Greek yogurt

½ tsp chili powder

2 tbsp garam masala

2 green chilies, sliced

1 bunch cilantro, chopped

Directions and Total Time: approx. 25 minutes

Take a pot, add water and bring it to a boil. Add pork and blanch for 4 minutes, remove and keep aside. Take a kadai, melt ghee, ginger, garlic, onions and saute for 5 minutes till they caramelize. Mix tomatoes and curd in it. Add chillies and garam masala. Stir well and cook for 12 minutes. Add coriander and green chillies to it. Take pork masala and serve with kouli rice.

Per serving: Cal 359; Net Carbs 4.2g; Fat 30g; Protein 38g

Pork Tenderloin and Pears

Preparation time: 10 minutes

Cooking time: 28 minutes

Servings: 4

Ingredients:

3 tablespoons olive oil

2 garlic cloves, minced

1 tablespoon thyme, chopped

1 and ½ pounds pork tenderloin

3 shallots, cut into medium wedges

3 pears, cored and quartered

4 tablespoons ghee, melted

1 and ½ cups chicken stock

¾ cup pear juice, unsweetened

Directions:

Take a bowl and toss oil, garlic, thyme, pear, shallots in it and mix. Heat a pan over medium high heat and add the tenderloin. Brown for 5 minutes and keep aside in a baking dish. Place in the oven and cook at 425 degrees F for 10 minutes and remove to plates. Add ghee to the same pan and heat it. Add stock and pear juice. Stir and cook for 5 minutes. Drizzle over the pork, shallots and serve.

Nutrition: calories 351, fat 3, fiber 6, carbs 15, protein 20

Green Pork Bake

Ingredients for 4 servings

1 lb ground pork

1 onion, chopped 1 garlic clove, minced

½ lb green beans, chopped

Salt and black pepper to taste

1 zucchini, sliced

¼ cup heavy cream

5 eggs

½ cup Monterey Jack cheese, grated

Directions and Total Time: approx. 50 minutes

Take a bowl and mix peas, ground pork, onion, garlic, black pepper and salt. Place the meat mixture in the bottom of a small greased baking dish. Place zucchini slices on top. Take another bowl and combine eggs, heavy cream, Monterey Jack cheese. Pour this mixture over the zucchini layer and bake for 40 minutes at 360 F until the edges and top are browned.

Per serving: Cal 445; Net Carbs 5.9g; Fat 31g; Protein 29g

Pork Tenderloin and Colored Peppers

Preparation time: 10 minutes

Cooking time: 22 minutes

Servings: 4

Ingredients:

1 pound pork tenderloin, trimmed and cut into medallions

A pinch of salt and black pepper

1 and ½ teaspoons rosemary, chopped

1 tablespoon olive oil

3 garlic cloves, minced

1 red bell pepper, cut into strips

1 yellow bell pepper, cut into strips

2 teaspoons balsamic vinegar

Directions:

Take a pan and heat it with oil on medium high temperature. Add pork, salt and pepper to it, stir and cook for 5 minutes. Add garlic, red and yellow bell peppers and rosemary and cook for 5 minutes. Add vinegar and cook for another 10 minutes. Transfer everything to plates and serve.

Nutrition: calories 300, fat 11, fiber 4, carbs 12, protein 18

Prosciutto Dish

Ingredients for 4 servings

4 prosciutto slices, cut into thirds

2 cups grated mozzarella

2 tbsp cream cheese, softened

½ cup almond flour

1 egg, beaten

⅓ cup tomato sauce

⅓ cup sliced mozzarella

6 fresh basil leaves, to serve

Directions and Total Time: approx. 40 minutes

Preheat the oven to 380 F. Line a dish pan with parchment paper. Microwave mozzarella cheese and 2 tbsp of cream cheese for 1 minute. Mix egg

and almond flour. Spread this mixture on a dish pan and bake for 20 minutes. Spread the tomato sauce over the crust. Arrange the mozzarella slices and then the prosciutto over the sauce. Bake again until the cheese melts. Remove and serve topped with basil.

Per serving: Cal 209; Net Carbs 4.5g; Fat 11g; Protein 19g

Pork and Scallions

Preparation time: 10 minutes

Cooking time: 6 minutes

Servings: 4

Ingredients:

1 pound pork tenderloin, cut into strips

1/3 cup chicken stock

¼ cup orange juice

2 tablespoons coconut aminos

1 teaspoon garlic sauce

A pinch of salt and black pepper

Cooking spray

1 and ½ teaspoons olive oil

2 cups carrots, cut into matchsticks

¼ cup water

2 teaspoons ginger, grated

¼ cup green onions, chopped

Directions:

Take a bowl and toss the pork, aminos, orange juice, garlic sauce, salt and pepper together. Heat a pan over medium high heat, grease it with cooking spray and add the pork. And cook each side and take out in a bowl. Heat the same pan on medium high heat and add water, ginger, carrots, onions and oranges and mix. Stir and cook for 5 minutes. Toss the pork in the pan, cook for another 2 minutes, divide and serve.

Nutrition: calories 288, fat 10, fiber 8, carbs 15, protein 22

Pork Soup

Preparation time: 10 minutes

Cooking time: 15 minutes

Servings: 4

Ingredients:

1 cup yellow onion, chopped

Cooking spray

2/3 cup green bell pepper, chopped

1 tablespoon garlic, minced

1 jalapeno pepper, chopped

1 pound pork tenderloin, cubed

2 cups chicken stock

2 teaspoons chili powder

1 teaspoon cumin, ground

A pinch of salt and black pepper

14 ounces canned tomatoes, chopped

2 tablespoons cilantro, chopped

Directions:

Heat a pot over medium-high heat with cooking spray. Add bell pepper, onion, garlic and jalapeno and stir and cook for 3 minutes. Stir in the stock, pork, cumin, chilli, salt, pepper and tomatoes, cover the pot and cook at a simmer for 12 minutes. Add coriander and cook for 5 minutes, remove in a bowl and serve.

Nutrition: calories 312, fat 3, fiber 6, carbs 12, protein 22

Gingery Pork Stir-Fry

Ingredients for 4 servings

2 tbsp coconut oil

1 ½ lb pork tenderloin

1 green bell pepper, diced

1 small red onion, diced

1/3 cup walnuts

1 tbsp freshly grated ginger

3 garlic cloves, minced

1 tsp olive oil

1 habanero pepper, minced

2 tbsp tamari sauce

Salt and black pepper to taste

Directions and Total Time: approx. 25 minutes

Take the pork and cut it into strips. Take a pan, heat coconut oil in it, add pork, salt and pepper and cook for 10 minutes. Shift to one side of the wok and add onion, walnuts, ginger, bell pepper, garlic, olive oil and habanero pepper. Cook the onion until soft. Season with tamari sauce. Fry for 2 minutes until well combined. Serve with cauliflower rice.

Per serving: Cal 318; Net Carbs 4.8g; Fat 16g; Protein 41g

Beef

Bell Pepper & Beef Sausage Frittata

Ingredients for 4 servings

12 whole eggs

1 cup sour cream

1 tbsp butter

2 red bell peppers, chopped

12 oz ground beef sausage

¼ cup shredded cheddar

Directions and Total Time: approx. 60 minutes

Preheat the oven to 350 F. Take a blender and break eggs in it, add salt, sour cream and pepper. Process on low speed until all ingredients are well mixed. and keep aside. Melt the butter in a large skillet over medium heat. Add bell pepper and cook until soft and keep aside. Add the beef sausage and cook for 10 minutes until browned. Place the beef in the bottom of the pan, spread the bell peppers on top, pour the egg mixture all over, and top with the cheddar cheese. Place the pan in the oven and bake until the cheese melts. Remove the frittata and serve hot with a nutty spinach salad.

Per serving: Cal 617; Net Carbs 5g; Fat 50g; Protein 33g

Chili Zucchini Beef Lasagna

Ingredients for 4 servings

½ cup Pecorino Romano cheese

4 yellow zucchini, sliced

Salt and black pepper to taste

1 tbsp lard

½ lb ground beef

1 tsp garlic powder

1 tsp onion powder

2 tbsp coconut flour

1 ½ cups grated mozzarella

2 cups crumbled goat cheese

1 large egg

2 cups marinara sauce

1 tbsp Italian herb seasoning

¼ tsp red chili flakes

¼ cup fresh basil leaves

Directions and Total Time: approx. 55 minutes

Preheat the oven to 375 F. Take a pan, melt the fat in it and cook the beef and set aside. In a bowl, combine the onion powder, coconut flour, garlic powder, salt, pepper, mozzarella cheese, goat cheese, half of the pecarino cheese and egg. Mix in the chili flakes marinara and Italian herb seasoning sauce. Arrange a layer of zucchini in a greased baking dish and spread 1/4 of the marinara sauce on top. and spread 1/4 of the egg mixture on top. Process again and top with remaining peccareno cheese. Bake in the oven for 20 minutes. Garnish with basil and serve.

Per serving: Cal 608; Net Carbs 5.5g; Fat 37g; Protein 52g

Tarragon Beef Meatloaf

Ingredients for 4 servings

2 lb ground beef

3 tbsp flaxseed meal

2 large eggs

2 tbsp olive oil

1 lemon, zested

¼ cup chopped tarragon

¼ cup chopped oregano

4 garlic cloves, minced

Directions and Total Time: approx. 70 minutes

Preheat the oven to 400 F. Grease a loaf pan with cooking spray. Take a bowl and mix salt, pepper, beef and flaxseed meal in it. and keep aside. In another bowl, whisk together the olive oil, eggs, lemon zest, oregano, tarragon and garlic. Pour the mixture over the beef mixture and combine evenly. Spoon the meat mixture into the pan and press down. Bake in the oven for 1 hour. Garnish with lemon wedges and serve with curry rice.

Per serving: Cal 631; Net Carbs 2.8g; Fat 38g; Protein 64g

Broccoli Beef Bake with Pancetta

Ingredients for 4 servings

1 large broccoli head, cut into florets

6 slices pancetta, chopped

2 tbsp olive oil

1 lb ground beef

2 tbsp butter

1 cup coconut cream

2 oz cream cheese, softened

1 ¼ cups grated cheddar

¼ cup chopped scallions

Directions and Total Time: approx. 55 minutes

Preheat the oven to 300 F. Boil water in a pot. Add broccoli and blanch for 3-4 minutes. Drain and keep aside. Fry the pancetta on both sides and keep aside in a plate. Heat olive oil in a pot and cook the beef until brown and set aside. Take a bowl, add cream cheese, coconut cream, butter, 2 thirds of

cheddar cheese, pepper and salt and stir for 5 minutes. Remove the broccoli florets to a baking dish and pour the cream mixture over them. Bake for another 30 minutes until the cheese is melted.

Per serving: Cal 854; Net Carbs 7.3g; Fat 69g; Protein 51g

Slow-Cooked BBQ Beef Sliders

Ingredients for 4 servings

4 zero carb hamburger buns, halved

3 lb chuck roast, boneless

1 tsp onion powder

2 tsp garlic powder

1 tbsp smoked paprika

2 tbsp tomato paste

¼ cup white vinegar

2 tbsp tamari sauce

½ cup bone broth

¼ cup melted butter

Salt and black pepper to taste

¼ cup baby spinach

4 slices cheddar cheese

Directions and Total Time: approx. 12 hours 25 minutes

Cut the beef into two pieces. Take a small bowl and mix together the onion, salt and pepper, garlic powder and paprika. Apply this mixture on the beef. In another bowl, mix vinegar, tamari sauce, chicken stock, tomato paste and melted butter. Add beef on it and cook for 6 hours. After the beef is cooked, cut it into two pieces. Divide the spinach over each bun, spoon the meat on top and add a slice of cheese. Cover and serve immediately.

Per serving: Cal 648; Net Carbs 17.6g; Fat 27g; Protein 72g

Roasted Beef Stacks with Cabbage

Ingredients for 6 servings

1 head canon cabbage, shredded

1 lb chuck steak, sliced thinly across the grain

3 tbsp coconut flour

¼ cup olive oil

2 tsp Italian mixed herb blend

½ cup bone broth

Directions and Total Time: approx. 55 minutes

Preheat the oven to 400 F. Add salt, pepper and coconut flour to a zipper bag. Mix and add the beef pieces. Seal the bag and shake to coat. Grease a baking sheet with olive oil and pile the cabbage. Sprinkle with salt and pepper and drizzle with 2 tablespoons of olive oil. Dip the beef strips in the coconut flour and shake off the excess flour. Place beef strips on top of each cabbage mound for 2-3 minutes. Sprinkle with Italian herb mixture and drizzle again with olive oil. After roasting for 30 minutes, remove the pan. Return to the oven and roast until the beef is cooked through.

Per serving: Cal 222; Net Carbs 1.5g; Fat 14g; Protein 18g

Savory Portobello Beef Burgers

Ingredients for 6 servings

6 large Portobello caps, destemmed and rinsed

1 lb ground beef

Salt and black pepper to taste

1 tbsp Worcestershire sauce

1 tbsp coconut oil

6 slices Monterey Jack

6 lettuce leaves

6 large tomato slices

¼ cup mayonnaise

Directions and Total Time: approx. 30 minutes

Take a bowl and combine the beef, Worcestershire sauce, salt and pepper. Mold the meat into 6 patties with your hands and set aside. Take a medium pan and heat coconut oil in it. Place the portobello in the caps and cook for 5 minutes until soft. Remove in a plate. Cook beef patties in skillet until browned, 10 minutes. Place the cheese slices on top of the beef and let it melt. Divide the lettuce on top, tomato slices, and top with mayo to serve.

Per serving: Cal 332; Net Carbs 0.7g; Fat 22g; Protein 29g

Spicy Enchilada Beef Stuffed Peppers

Ingredients for 6 servings

6 bell peppers, deseeded

1 ½ tbsp olive oil

3 tbsp butter, softened

½ white onion, chopped

3 cloves garlic, minced

2 ½ lb ground beef

3 tsp enchilada seasoning

1 cup cauliflower rice

¼ cup grated cheddar cheese

Sour cream for serving

Directions and Total Time: approx. 70 minutes

Preheat the oven to 400 F. Take a pan, melt butter in it and fry onion and garlic in it. Stir in beef, enchilada seasoning, salt and pepper. Mix the kouli rice until smooth. Spoon the mixture into the peppers and divide the cheddar cheese on top. Place the stuffed peppers in a baking dish and bake for 40 minutes. Drop generous dollops of sour cream over the peppers to serve.

Per serving: Cal 409; Net Carbs 4g; Fat 21g; Protein 45g

Spicy Beef Lettuce Wraps

Ingredients for 4 servings

1 lb chuck steak, sliced thinly against the grain

3 tbsp ghee, divided

1 large white onion, chopped

2 garlic cloves, minced

1 jalapeño pepper, chopped

2 tsp red curry powder

1 cup cauliflower rice

8 small lettuce leaves

¼ cup sour cream for topping

Directions and Total Time: approx. 20 minutes

Take a large pan and melt 2 tbsp ghee in it. Season the beef and cook for 10 minutes and set aside. Fry onion in it for 4 minutes. Add in the salt, pepper and garlic and jalapeño. Add remaining ghee, beef and curry leaves and cook for 5 minutes. Also stir the flower rice. Add salt and pepper to taste. Lay out the lettuce leaves on a lean flat surface and spoon the beef mixture onto the middle part of the leaves, about 3 tbsp per leaf. Divide sour cream on top, wrap the leaves, and serve.

Per serving: Cal 298; Net Carbs 3.3g; Fat 18g; Protein 27g

Sunday Beef Fathead

Ingredients for 4 servings

2 tbsp cream cheese, softened

6 oz shredded cheese

¾ cup almond flour

1 egg

1 tsp plain vinegar

2 tbsp butter

8 oz ground beef sausage

¼ cup tomato sauce

½ tsp dried basil

4 ½ oz shredded mozzarella

Directions and Total Time: approx. 45 minutes

Preheat oven to 400 F. Line a pizza pan with parchment paper. Melt cream and mozzarella cheeses in a skillet while stirring until evenly combined. Turn off the heat and mix the vinegar, almond flour and salt and let it cool slightly. Spread the mixture on the pizza pan. Cover with another parchment paper and using a rolling pin, smoothen the dough into a circle. Take off the parchment paper on top, prick the dough all over with a fork, and bake for 10 to 15 minutes until golden brown. Melt the butter in a pan and fry the sausages for 10 minutes and turn off the heat. Spread the tomato sauce over the crust and top with the meat, mozzarella cheese and basil. Bake in the oven for 10 minutes. Take out the pizza and slice and serve.

Per serving: Cal 361; Net Carbs 0.8g; Fat 21g; Protein 37g

Lemon & Spinach Cheeseburgers

Ingredients for 4 servings

1 large tomato, sliced into 4 pieces and deseeded

1 lb ground beef

½ cup chopped cilantro

1 lemon, zested and juiced

Salt and black pepper to taste

1 tsp garlic powder

2 tbsp hot chili puree

16 large spinach leaves

4 tbsp mayonnaise

1 medium red onion, sliced

¼ cup grated Parmesan

1 avocado, halved, sliced

Directions and Total Time: approx. 15 minutes

Heat grill to high temperature. Take a bowl and add coriander, beef, lemon juice, salt, pepper, garlic powder and chili puree. Put on gloves and mix until the mixture is smooth. Make 3 patties from the mixture and grill for 3 minutes. Transfer to a serving plate. Lay 2 spinach leaves side to side in 4 portions on a clean flat surface. Place a beef patty on each, spread a tbsp of mayo on top of the meat, add a slice of tomato and onion, sprinkle with some Parmesan cheese, and divide avocado on top. Cover with 2 pieces of spinach leaves each. Serve the burgers with cream cheese sauce.

Per serving: Cal 310; Net Carbs 6.5g; Fat 16g; Protein 29g

Herby Beef Meatballs

Ingredients for 4 servings

3 lb ground beef

1 red onion, finely chopped

2 red bell peppers, chopped

3 garlic cloves, minced

2 tbsp melted butter

1 tsp dried basil

2 tbsp tamari sauce

Salt and black pepper to taste

1 tbsp dried rosemary

3 tbsp olive oil

Directions and Total Time: approx. 30 minutes

Preheat the oven to 400 F and grease a baking sheet with cooking spray. Take a bowl and mix bell pepper, beef, onion, butter, tamari sauce, garlic, basil, salt, pepper and rosemary. Form 1 inch meatballs from the mixture and place on a greased baking sheet. Drizzle the beef with olive oil and bake in the oven for 20 minutes. Serve.

Per serving: Cal 618; Net Carbs 2.5g; Fat 33g; Protein 74g

Peanut Zucchini & Beef Pad Thai

Ingredients for 4 servings

2 ½ lb chuck steak, sliced thinly against the grain

1 tsp crushed red pepper flakes

¼ tsp freshly pureed garlic

¼ tsp freshly ground ginger

Salt and black pepper to taste

2 tbsp peanut oil

3 large eggs, lightly beaten

1/3 cup beef broth

3 ¼ tbsp peanut butter

2 tbsp tamari sauce

1 tbsp white vinegar

½ cup chopped green onions

2 garlic cloves, minced

4 zucchinis, spiralized

½ cup bean sprouts

½ cup crushed peanuts

Directions and Total Time: approx. 35 minutes

Take a bowl and mix ginger, garlic, salt and pepper in it. Add beef and toss to coat. Heat groundnut oil in a pan and cook the beef for 10 minutes and remove to a plate. Add eggs to the skillet and scramble and keep aside. Combine peanut butter, broth, tamari sauce, vinegar, green onions, garlic, and red pepper flakes over medium heat. Mix and simmer for 5 minutes until well combined. Stir in the zucchini, beef and bean sprouts and eggs. Serve.

Per serving: Cal 425; Net Carbs 3.3g; Fat 40g; Protein 70g

Beef Taco

Ingredients for 4 servings

2 cups shredded mozzarella

2 tbsp cream cheese, softened

1 egg

¾ cup almond flour

1 lb ground beef

2 tsp taco seasoning

½ cup cheese sauce

1 cup grated cheddar cheese

1 cup chopped lettuce

1 tomato, diced

¼ cup sliced black olives

1 cup sour cream for topping

Directions and Total Time: approx. 45 minutes

Preheat the oven to 390 F and line a pizza pan with parchment paper. Microwave the mozzarella and cream cheese for 1 minute. Remove and mix with almond and egg batter. Spread the mixture on the pan and bake for 20 minutes. Stir in taco seasoning; salt and pepper. Spread the cheese sauce over the crust. Add cheddar cheese, lettuce, tomato and black olives. Bake for 5 minutes. Remove the pizza and serve with sour cream on top.

Per serving: Cal 590; Net Carbs 7.9g; Fat 29g; Protein 64g

Mushroom & Bell Pepper Beef Skewers

Ingredients for 4 servings

2 cups cremini mushrooms, halved

2 yellow bell peppers, deseeded and cut into squares

2 lb tri-tip steak, cubed

2 tbsp coconut oil

1 tbsp tamari sauce

3 limes, juiced

1 tbsp ginger powder

½ tsp ground cumin

Directions and Total Time: approx. 1 hour 25 minutes

Take a bowl and mix coconut oil, lemon juice, tamari sauce, salt, pepper and cumin seeds in it. Add the mushrooms, beef, and bell pepper and toss to coat. Cover the bowl with plastic wrap and marinate for 1 hour. Heat grill to high temperature. Remove the plastic wrap and thread the mushrooms, beef, and bell pepper onto each skewer in that order until the ingredients are gone. Grill the skewers for 5 minutes on each side. Remove to a plate, garnish with sesame seeds, and serve hot with steamed cauliflower rice or braised asparagus.

Per serving: Cal 383; Net Carbs 3.2g; Fat 17g; Protein 51g

Hot Beef & Cauli Rice with Cashew Nuts

Ingredients for 4 servings

3 tbsp olive oil

1 ½ lb chuck steak

2 large eggs, beaten

1 tbsp avocado oil

1 red onion, finely chopped

½ cup chopped bell peppers

½ cup green beans, chopped

3 garlic cloves, minced

4 cups cauliflower rice

¼ cup coconut aminos

1 cup toasted cashew nuts

1 tbsp toasted sesame seeds

Directions and Total Time: approx. 25 minutes

Take a pan and heat 2 tablespoons of olive oil on medium heat. Season the beef with salt and pepper and cook in oil and set aside. Add eggs and scramble and keep aside. Add the remaining olive oil and avocado oil to the pan. Mix bell pepper, peas, onion and garlic. Stir in coconut aminos, cauli rice until evenly combined. Mix eggs, beef and cashews and cook for 5 minutes. Turn off the heat and serve hot.

Per serving: Cal 500; Net Carbs 3.2g; Fat 32; Protein 44g

Coconut Beef with Mushroom & Olive Sauce

Ingredients for 4 servings

¼ cup button mushrooms, sliced

3 tbsp unsalted butter

1 yellow onion, chopped

4 rib-eye steaks

1/3 cup coconut milk

2 tbsp coconut cream

1/2 tsp dried thyme

2 tbsp chopped parsley

3 tbsp black olives, sliced

Directions and Total Time: approx. 30 minutes

Take a large pan, melt 2 tbsp of butter on medium heat, add mushrooms and saute. Stir the onion and cook and set aside. Sprinkle salt and pepper over the beef. Melt the remaining butter in a pan and cook the beef for 10 minutes on both sides. Add the onion and mushrooms to the pan and add the coconut cream, milk, thyme and 1 tablespoon of oats. Stir and boil for 2-3 minutes. Mix in the olives and turn off the heat. Serve.

Per serving: Cal 639; Net Carbs 1.9g; Fat 39g; Protein 69g

Maple BBQ Rib Steak

Ingredients for 4 servings

2 lb rib steak, membrane removed

2 tbsp avocado oil

3 tbsp maple syrup, sugar-free

3 tbsp barbecue dry rub

Directions and Total Time: approx. 2 hours 40 minutes

Preheat the oven to 300 F and line a baking sheet with aluminum foil. Take a bowl, mix maple syrup, avocado oil and pour the mixture over the meat and sprinkle and rub the BBQ all over the meat. Place the ribs on a baking sheet and bake until crisp. Serve with green beans.

Per serving: Cal 490; Net Carbs 1.8g; Fat 26g; Protein 49g

Burgers

Ingredients for 4 servings

1 pound ground beef

½ tsp onion powder

½ tsp garlic powder

2 tbsp ghee

1 tsp Dijon mustard

4 zero carb burger buns

¼ cup mayonnaise

1 tsp Sriracha sauce

4 tbsp slaw

Salt and black pepper to taste

Directions and Total Time: approx. 15 minutes

Combine onion powder, mustard, salt, garlic powder, beef, pepper. 4 Prepare the burgers. Take a kadai, melt ghee in it and cook for 2 minutes on each side. Serve on a bun topped with mayonnaise, sriracha sauce, and slaw.

Per serving: Cal 664; Net Carbs 7.9g; Fat 55g; Protein 39g

Beef & Shiitake Mushroom Stir-Fry

Ingredients for 4 servings

2 cups shiitake mushrooms, halved

2 sprigs rosemary, leaves extracted

1 green bell pepper, chopped

1 lb chuck steak

4 slices prosciutto, chopped

1 tbsp coconut oil

1 tbsp freshly pureed garlic

Directions and Total Time: approx. 30 minutes

Cut the chuck stick into thin slices and sprinkle with salt and pepper. Heat a kadai on medium heat. Fry the prosciutto until crisp and set aside. Melt coconut oil in a pan and cook the beef. Remove the prosciutto plate. Add mushrooms and bell peppers and sauté until softened, 5 minutes. Stir in the prosciutto, beef, rosemary and garlic. Season to taste and cook for 5 minutes. Serve with buttered green beans.

Per serving: Cal 231; Net Carbs 2.1g; Fat 12g; Protein 27g

Garlicky Beef with Creamy Curry Sauce

Ingredients for 4 servings

2 tbsp ghee

4 large rib-eye steak

2 garlic cloves, minced

½ cup chopped brown onion

1 green bell pepper, sliced

1 red bell pepper, sliced

2 long red chilies, sliced

1 cup beef stock

1 cup coconut milk

1 tbsp Thai green curry paste

1 lime, juiced

3 tbsp chopped cilantro

Directions and Total Time: approx. 40 minutes

Take a pan and melt 1 tbsp of ghee on medium heat and add beef, salt and pepper and cook on each side. Remove in a plate. Take a kadai and add the remaining ghee in it and saute the onion. Saute the red chillies and bell peppers until soft. Add curry paste, coconut milk, beef stock and lemon juice and simmer for 5 minutes. Return the beef to the sauce and cook for 10 minutes. Place the pan in the oven. Cook under the broiler for another 4 minutes. Garnish with flowers and cilantro and serve with rice.

Per serving: Cal 644; Net Carbs 2.6g; Fat 35g; Protein 72g

Walnut Beef Skillet with Brussel Sprouts

Ingredients for 4 servings

¼ cup toasted walnuts, chopped

1 ½ cups Brussel sprouts, halved

2 tbsp avocado oil

1 garlic clove, minced

½ white onion, chopped

Salt and black pepper to taste

1 lb ground beef

1 bok choy, quartered

2 tbsp chopped scallions

1 tbsp black sesame seeds

Directions and Total Time: approx. 30 minutes

Take a pan and heat 1 tbsp of avocado oil in it. Add onion and garlic and saute. Stir in the ground beef and cook for 5 minutes. Add the Brussels sprouts, bok choy, walnuts, scallions and salt and pepper. Saute for 4 minutes. Dish into a serving plate and serve with low carb bread.

Per serving: Cal 302; Net Carbs 3.1g; Fat 18g; Protein 29g

Easy Pressure-Cooked Shredded Beef

Ingredients for 4 servings

3 tbsp coconut oil

1 large white onion, chopped

3 garlic cloves, minced

1 cup shredded red cabbage

1 lemon, zested and juiced

1 tsp dried Italian herb blend

1 ½ tbsp balsamic vinegar

½ cup beef broth

2 lb chuck steak

Salt and black pepper to taste

Directions and Total Time: approx. 45 minutes

Select the saute mode on the pressure cooker. Heat coconut oil and saute garlic, cabbage and onion in it for 2 minutes. Stir in lemon juice, lemon zest, Italian herb blend, balsamic vinegar, salt, and pepper. Mix in the broth. Sprinkle salt and pepper over the meat. Place in the cooker and close the lid. Select manual mode on high for 30 minutes. When the timer is up, release the natural pressure, then release the quick pressure to release any remaining steam and open the lid. Shred the meat using two forks. Select Sauté to reduce the sauce, 5 minutes, and then spoon the beef over a bed of zucchini noodles with the sauce. Serve.

Per serving: Cal 652; Net Carbs 5.8g; Fat 49g; Protein 44g

Easy Beef Burger Bake

Ingredients for 4 servings

¼ cup shredded Monterey Jack cheese

1 tbsp butter

1 lb ground beef

1 garlic clove, minced

1 medium red onion, chopped

2 tomatoes

1 tbsp dried basil

Salt and black pepper to taste

2 eggs

2 tbsp tomato paste

1 cup coconut cream

Directions and Total Time: approx. 35 minutes

Preheat the oven to 400 F. Take a large kadai, melt butter in it, add beef and cook. Saute garlic and onion. Mix basil, tomatoes, salt and pepper. Add 2/3 of the Monterey Jack cheese and stir to melt. Take a bowl and whisk it with tomato paste, beaten eggs, salt and coconut cream. Place the beef mixture on a baking sheet and spread the egg mixture over it. Bake for another 20 minutes with remaining cheese and serve.

Per serving: Cal 469; Net Carbs 4.5g; Fat 34g; Protein 33g

Awesome Zucchini Boats Stuffed with Beef

Ingredients for 4 servings4

2 zucchinis

2 tbsp butter

1 lb ground beef

1 red bell pepper, chopped

2 garlic cloves, minced

1 shallot, finely chopped

2 tbsp taco seasoning

½ cup finely chopped parsley

1 tbsp olive oil

1¼ cups shredded cheddar

Directions and Total Time: approx. 50 minutes

Preheat the oven to 400 F. Grease a baking sheet with cooking spray. Cut the zucchini in half and scoop out the pulp to make 4 vegetable boats. Chop the meat. Take a pan, melt the butter on medium heat and cook the beef, stirring frequently. Add garlic, bell pepper, pulp, garlic, shallot, taco seasoning and cook until soft. Place the boats on the baking sheet with the open side up. Divide the eggs into the beef mixture. Drizzle with olive oil. Bake until cheese melts. Plate the boats and serve hot with a tangy lettuce salad.

Per serving: Cal 423; Net Carbs 2.9g; Fat 29g; Protein 35g

Sage Beef Meatloaf with Pecans

Ingredients for 4 servings

2 tbsp olive oil

1 white onion, finely chopped

1 ½ lb ground beef

½ cup coconut cream

½ cup shredded Parmesan

1 egg, lightly beaten

1 tbsp dried sage

4 tbsp toasted pecans, chopped

Salt and black pepper to taste

6 bacon slices

Directions and Total Time: approx. 45 minutes

Preheat the oven to 400 F. Heat olive oil in a pan. Fry onion in it. Take a bowl and mix together the onion, coconut cream, ground beef, Parmesan cheese, eggs, sage, pecans, salt and pepper. Make a loaf and wrap it in a piece of bacon and place it on a greased baking sheet with toothpicks and bake for 25 minutes. Slice and serve.

Per serving: Cal 617; Net Carbs 6.6g; Fat 43g; Protein 48g

Tangy Cabbage & Beef Bowl with Creamy Blue Cheese

Ingredients for 4 servings

3 tbsp butter

1 canon cabbage, shredded

1 tsp onion powder

1 tsp garlic powder

2 tsp dried oregano

1 tbsp red wine vinegar

1 ½ lb ground beef

1 cup coconut cream

¼ cup blue cheese

½ cup fresh parsley, chopped

Directions and Total Time: approx. 25 minutes

Take a pan, melt 1 tbsp of butter in it and saute oregano, salt, pepper, onion and garlic powder, cabbage and vinegar. Keep aside. Take a pan, melt 1 tablespoon of butter in it and cook the beef, stirring frequently. Stir in coconut cream and blue cheese for 4 minutes until cheese melts. Dish into serving bowls with low carb bread.

Per serving: Cal 542; Net Carbs 4.2g; Fat 41g; Protein 41g

Cheesy Tomato Beef Tart

Ingredients for 4 servings

2 tbsp olive oil

1 small brown onion, chopped

1 garlic clove, finely chopped

2 lb ground beef

1 tbsp Italian mixed herbs

4 tbsp tomato paste

4 tbsp coconut flour

¾ cup almond flour

4 tbsp flaxseeds

1 tsp baking powder

3 tbsp coconut oil, melted

1 egg

¼ cup ricotta, crumbled

¼ cup shredded cheddar

Directions and Total Time: approx. 1 hour 30 minutes

Preheat the oven to 350 F. Line pie dish with parchment paper and grease with cooking spray; Set aside. Take a large pan and heat oil on medium heat. Saute onion and garlic in it until soft. Add beef and cook. Season with herbs, salt and pepper. Stir in the tomato paste and half a cup of water and reduce the heat. Boil for 20 minutes; Set aside. Add baking powder, flour, flaxseed, salt, eggs, coconut oil and 3 tablespoons water to a food processor. Mix until a dough is formed. Spread batter in pie pan and bake for 10 minutes. Take a small bowl, mix the ricotta and cheddar cheese and spread the cheese on top. Bake for 30 minutes until cheese is melted. Remove pie, let cool 3 minutes, slice and serve with green salad and garlic vinaigrette. Preheat the oven to 350 F. Line pie dish with parchment paper and grease with cooking spray; Set aside. Take a large pan and heat oil on medium heat. Saute onion and garlic in it until soft. Add beef and cook. Season with herbs, salt and pepper. Stir in the tomato paste and half a cup of water and reduce the heat. Boil for 20 minutes; Set aside. Add baking powder, flour, flaxseed, salt, eggs, coconut oil and 3 tablespoons water to a food processor. Mix until a dough is formed. Spread batter in pie pan and bake for 10 minutes. Take a small bowl, mix the ricotta and cheddar cheese and spread the cheese on top. Bake for 30 minutes until cheese is melted. Remove pie, let cool 3 minutes, slice and serve with green salad and garlic vinaigrette.

Per serving: Cal 603; Net Carbs 2.3g; Fat 39g; Protein 57g

Olive & Pesto Beef Casserole with Goat Cheese

Ingredients for 4 servings

2 tbsp ghee

1 ½ lb ground beef

Salt and black pepper to taste

3 oz pitted green olives

5 oz goat cheese, crumbled

1 garlic clove, minced

3 oz basil pesto

1¼ cups coconut cream

Directions and Total Time: approx. 45 minutes

Preheat the oven to 400 F and grease a casserole dish with cooking spray. Take a kadai, melt ghee in it and cook the beef. Spread the beef in the bottom of the casserole dish. Top with olives, goat cheese and garlic. Take a bowl and mix coconut cream and pesto cream in it and pour this mixture over the beef. Bake for 20 minutes and serve with a green salad.

Per serving: Cal 656; Net Carbs 4g; Fat 51g; Protein 47g

Maple Jalapeño Beef Plate

Ingredients for 4 servings

1 lb ribeye steak, sliced into ¼-inch strips

2 tsp sugar-free maple syrup

Salt and black pepper to taste

1 tbsp coconut flour

1/2 tsp xanthan gum

½ cup olive oil, for frying

1 tbsp coconut oil

1 tsp freshly pureed ginger

1 clove garlic, minced

1 red chili, minced

4 tbsp tamari sauce

1 tsp sesame oil

1 tsp fish sauce

2 tbsp white wine vinegar

1 tsp hot sauce

1 small bok choy, quartered

½ jalapeño, sliced into rings

1 tbsp toasted sesame seeds

1 scallion, chopped

Directions and Total Time: approx. 40 minutes

Sprinkle the beef with salt and pepper and toss with the coconut flour and xanthan gum and set aside. Take a pan, heat olive oil on medium heat and fry the beef. Heat coconut oil in a pan and fry red chillies, bok choy and garlic in it. Cook by mixing in sesame oil, fish sauce, tamari sauce, vinegar, hot sauce and maple syrup. Add beef and cook further. Spoon into bowl, top with jalapeños, scallion and sesame seeds. Serve.

Per serving: Cal 507; Net Carbs 2.9g; Fat 43g; Protein 25g

Cheese & Beef Avocado Boats

Ingredients for 4 servings

4 tbsp avocado oil

1 lb ground beef

Salt and black pepper to taste

1 tsp onion powder

1 tsp cumin powder

1 tsp garlic powder

2 tsp taco seasoning

2 tsp smoked paprika

1 cup raw pecans, chopped

1 tbsp hemp seeds, hulled

7 tbsp shredded Monterey Jack

2 avocados, halved and pitted

1 medium tomato, sliced

¼ cup shredded iceberg lettuce

4 tbsp sour cream

4 tbsp shredded Monterey Jack

Directions and Total Time: approx. 30 minutes

Take a pan, heat half the avocado oil in it and cook the beef for 8 minutes. Season with onion powder, taco seasoning, paprika, garlic, cumin, salt and pepper. Add hemp and pecan seeds and saute. Fold in 3 tablespoons Monterey Jack cheese to melt. Spoon the filling into the avocado holes, top with 1-2 tomato slices, some lettuce, a tablespoon each of sour cream and the remaining Monterey Jack cheese, and serve immediately.

Per serving: Cal 840; Net Carbs 4g; Fat 70g; Protein 42g

Morning Beef Bowl

Ingredients for 4 servings

1 lb beef sirloin, cut into strips

¼ cup tamari sauce

2 tbsp lemon juice

3 tsp garlic powder

1 tbsp swerve sugar

1 cup coconut oil

6 garlic cloves, minced

1 lb cauliflower rice

2 tbsp olive oil

4 large eggs

2 tbsp chopped scallions

Directions and Total Time: approx. 35 min + chilling time

Take a bowl and add garlic powder, lemon juice, tamari sauce and swerve. Add the spices to the beef and place in a zipper bag. Mash well to coat. Refrigerate overnight. The next day, heat coconut oil in a pan and fry the beef till the meat is cooked. and keep aside. Saute the garlic. Mix until the kouli rice is soft. Season with salt and pepper and remove into 4 serving bowls and set aside. Wipe the pan clean and heat 1 tbsp olive oil in it. Crack two eggs and fry them. Place one egg on top of each bowl of cauliflower rice and fry the other 2 eggs with the remaining olive oil. Serve garnished with scallions.

Per serving: Cal 908; Net Carbs 5.1g; Fat 83g; Protein 34g

Rosemary Beef Meatza

Ingredients for 4 servings

1 ½ lb ground beef

Salt and black pepper to taste

1 large egg

1 tsp rosemary

1 tsp thyme

3 garlic cloves, minced

1 tsp basil

½ tbsp oregano

¾ cup low-carb tomato sauce

¼ cup shredded Parmesan

1 cup shredded Pepper Jack

1 cup shredded mozzarella

Directions and Total Time: approx. 30 minutes

Preheat the oven to 350 F. And grease the pizza pan with cooking spray. Take a bowl and combine the beef, salt, pepper, egg, basil, garlic, thyme, rosemary and oregano. Transfer the mixture to the pan. and flatten by hand to a thickness of two inches. Bake the beef for 20 minutes. Remove the tomato sauce and spread it on top. Sprinkle with mozzarella cheese, pepper jack and parmesan. Bake until cheese melts.

Per serving: Cal 319; Net Carbs 3.6g; Fat 10g; Protein

Recipes In Alphabetical Order

A

B

Bacon Stew with Cauliflower 129
Bacon Wrapped Sausages 113
Bacon and Lemon Thyme Muffins 24
Bacon, Cheese & Avocado Mug Cakes 8
Baked Chicken Nuggets 145
Baked Eggs with Sausage 42
Baked Tenderloin with Lime Chimichurri 174
Balsamic Chicken 147
Balsamic Steaks 101
Barbecue Baked Pork Chops 160
Basil Pork Meatballs in Tomato Sauce 172
Basil Prosciutto Pizza 175
Beef & Shiitake Mushroom Stir-Fry 202
Beef & Veggie Stew 131
Beef Curry 106
Beef Meatballs 99
Beef Meatloaf 32
Beef Salad 99
Beef Taco 200
Beef and Kale pan 103
Beef and Radish Stew 102
Beef, Avocado and Eggs 28
Belgium Waffles with Cheese Spread 4
Bell Pepper & Beef Sausage Frittata 194
Bell Pepper & Cheese Frittata 28
Bell Pepper Noodles with Pork Avocado 176
Bell Peppers and Avocado Bowls 8
Berry Hemp seed Breakfast 13
Brazilian Moqueca (Shrimp Stew) 133
Breadless Breakfast Sandwich 16
Breakfast Bowl 6
Breakfast Bread 48
Breakfast Bread 8
Breakfast Broccoli Muffins 14
Breakfast Burger 4
Breakfast Casserole 39
Breakfast Cauliflower Mix 7
Breakfast Hash 34
Breakfast Muffins 11
Breakfast Muffins 49
Breakfast Pie 33
Breakfast Pork Bagel 18
Breakfast Skillet 37

C

Cheddar & Broccoli Soup 117
Cheddar & Turkey Meatball Salad 70
Cheddar Pork Burrito Bowl 158
Cheese & Beef Avocado Boats 207
Cheese Cream Soup with Chicken 92
Cheese and Oregano Muffins 27
Cheesy Beef Salad 68
Cheesy Chicken Soup with Spinach 93
Cheesy Coconut Cookies 12
Cheesy Mushrooms & Bacon Lettuce Rolls 160
Cheesy Pinwheels with Chicken 138
Cheesy Pork Casserole 104
Cheesy Pork Quiche 154
Cheesy Sausages in Creamy Onion Sauce 169
Cheesy Tomato Beef Tart 206
Cheesy Turkey Pan 97
Cheesy Zucchini Soup 60
Chia Bowls 46
Chia Pudding 38
Chicken And Shrimp 115
Chicken Breakfast Muffins 17
Chicken Breasts with Creamy Kale Sauce 144
Chicken Calzone 141
Chicken Dippers with Homemade Ketchup 147
Chicken Enchilada Soup 119
Chicken Enchilada Soup 53
Chicken Enchilada Soup 79
Chicken Gumbo 137
Chicken Kabobs with Celery Root Chips 149
Chicken Meatballs and Sauce 100
Chicken Meatloaf 143
Chicken Mushroom Soup 89
Chicken Noodle Soup 55
Chicken Pasta 148
Chicken Salad with Gorgonzola Cheese 70
Chicken Salad with Parmesan 58
Chicken Soup 105
Chicken Stew 102
Chicken Stew with Spinach 129
Chicken Stroganoff 136
Chicken Thighs with Mushrooms and Cheese 138
Chicken and Cabbage Stew 53
Chicken and Leeks Pan 97

Chicken and Peppers Mix 98
Chicken with Green Onion Sauce 145
Chicken with Sour Cream Sauce 136
Chicken "Ramen" Soup 54
Chicken, Avocado & Egg Bowls 62
Chicken-stuffed Avocados 146
Chicken-stuffed Mushrooms 146
Chili Beef Stew with Cauliflower Grits 130
Chili Omelet with Avocado 34
Chili Spinach and Beef Mix 34
Chili Tomatoes and Eggs 2
Chili Zucchini Beef Lasagna 194
Chilled Lemongrass & Avocado Soup 125
Chinese Tofu Soup 83
Chorizo & Cauliflower Soup 120
Chorizo & Cheese Frittata 27
Chorizo & Tomato Salad with Olives 79
Chorizo Egg Cups 36
Chorizo Smoky Pizza 177
Chorizo and Cauliflower Breakfast 43
Chorizo in Cabbage Sauce with Pine Nuts 151
Classic Egg Salad with Olives 57
Classic Greek Salad 75
Cobb Salad with Roquefort Dressing 54
Coconut Beef with Mushroom & Olive Sauce 201
Coconut Berries Bowls 45
Coconut Cream Pumpkin Soup 119
Coconut Curry Cauliflower Soup 95
Coconut Turkey Chili 128
Colby Cauliflower Soup with Pancetta Chips 127
Cold Green Beans and Avocado Soup 90
Crabmeat Frittata with Onion 29
Cranberry & Tempeh Broccoli Salad 81
Cream Soup with Avocado & Zucchini 82
Cream of Cauliflower & Leek Soup 96
Cream of Roasted Jalapeño Soup 97
Creamy Artichoke Soup 76
Creamy Asparagus Soup 94
Creamy Chicken Soup 119
Creamy Coconut Soup with Chicken 95
Creamy Eggs 13
Creamy Eggs and Asparagus 2
Creamy Leek & Salmon Soup 58

D

E

F

G

Jerk Pork Pot Roast 181
Juicy Chicken with Broccoli & Pine Nuts 145
Juicy Pork Chops with Parmesan 165

K

Kale & Broccoli Slaw with Bacon & Parmesan 60
Kale Frittata 49

L

Lazy Eggs with Feta Cheese 25
Leeks Breakfast Mix 47
Leeks and Eggs Mix 42
Lemon & Spinach Cheeseburgers 198
Lemon Garlic Mason Jar Salad 75
Lemony Greek Pork Tenderloin 163
Lettuce, Beet & Tofu Salad 81
Lime Turkey Soup 105
Lunch Green Beans Salad 108
Lunch Lobster Bisque 114
Lunch Spinach Rolls 106
Lunch Stew 115

M

Maple BBQ Rib Steak 201
Maple Jalapeño Beef Plate 207
Maple Pork with Spaghetti Squash 178
Maple Scallion Pork Bites 181
Marinated Fried Chicken 142
Meatball Soup 188
Meatballs And Pilaf 107
Meatless Club Salad 66

Mediterranean Artichoke Salad 63
Mediterranean Stuffed Chicken Breasts 142
Mexican Breakfast 30
Mexican Chicken Soup 141
Microwave Bacon Frittata 24
Mini Raspberry Tarts 18
Mint Avocado Chilled Soup 62
Mixed Green Salad 82
Mixed Mushroom Soup 124
Modern Greek Salad with Avocado 66
Monterey Jack & Sausage-Pepper Pizza 178
Morning Beef Bowl 208
Morning Chia Pudding 14
Morning Herbed Eggs 31
Mozzarella Baked Pork 165
Mushroom & Bell Pepper Beef Skewers 200
Mushroom & Cheese Lettuce Cups 21
Mushroom & Pork Casserole 167
Mushroom Cream Soup with Herbs 87
Mushroom Omelet 5
Mushroom Pork Meatballs with Parsnips 166

N

Nut Porridge with Strawberries 12
Nutmeg Pumpkin Soup 95
Nutritious Breakfast Salad 12
Nutty Breakfast Bowl 47
Nutty Breakfast Bowl 6

O

Olive & Pesto Beef Casserole with Goat Cheese 206
One–pot Roasted Chicken 144
Oven Baked Pork Chops with Salad 71

P

Q

R

S

Salmon Cakes 48
Salmon Frittata 41
Salmon Soup 116
Salmon Stew 56
Saucy Thai Pork Medallions 160
Sausage & Pesto Salad with Cheese 55
Sausage & Turnip Soup 90
Sausage And Pepper Soup 82
Sausage Cakes with Poached Eggs 31
Sausage Patties 40
Sausage Quiche 41
Sausage-Pepper Soup 80
Savory Jalapeño Pork Meatballs 169
Savory Pork Tacos 157
Savory Portobello Beef Burgers 196
Savory Waffles with Cheese & Tomato 7
Scottish Beef Stew 129
Scrambled Eggs 11
Scrambled Eggs with Tofu & Mushrooms 32
Seared Rump Steak Salad 67
Seasoned Hard Boiled Eggs 25
Seeded Morning Loaf 16
Serrano Ham Frittata with Salad 26
Sesame & Poppy Seed Bagels 11
Sesame Pork Meatballs 163
Shrimp Salad with Avocado 76
Shrimp and Bacon Breakfast 28
Shrimp and Eggs Mix 15
Shrimp and Eggs Mix 49
Shrimp and Olives Pan 26
Shrimp and Zucchini Pan 100
Simple Asparagus Lunch 111
Simple Breakfast Cereal 40
Simple Buffalo Wings 112
Simple Chicken Stir–fry 142
Simple Egg Porridge 40
Simple Halloumi Salad 114
Simple Lunch Apple Salad 110
Simple Shrimp Pasta 111
Simple Tomato Soup 113
Slow Cooked Ribs 185
Slow Cooked Sausage Soup with Beer 118
Slow-Cooked BBQ Beef Sliders 195

Smoked Mackerel Lettuce Cups 59
Smoked Paprika-Coconut Tenderloin 166
Smoked Salmon Breakfast 17
Smoked Salmon Salad 72
Smoked Salmon, Bacon & Egg Salad 56
South-American Shrimp Stew 134
Spiced Biscuits 13
Spiced Pumpkin Soup 78
Spicy Beef Lettuce Wraps 197
Spicy Enchilada Beef Stuffed Peppers 197
Spicy Frittata 43
Spicy Grilled Pork Spareribs 179
Spicy Halibut Tomato Soup 58
Spinach & Brussels Sprout Salad 57
Spinach & Feta Cheese Pancakes 5
Spinach & Kale Soup with Fried Collards 122
Spinach & Poached Egg Soup 121
Spinach Nests with Eggs & Cheese 19
Spinach Omelet 38
Spinach Pesto Eggs Mix 48
Spinach Salad with Goat Cheese & Nuts 65
Spinach Salad with Pancetta & Mustard 63
Spinach and Artichoke Chicken 143
Spinach and Cauliflower Pan 50
Spinach and Eggs Salad 10
Spinach and Watercress Salad 70
Spring Soup with Poached Egg 62
Spring Vegetable Soup 124
Stuffed Chicken Breasts 137
Summer Gazpacho with Cottage Cheese 83
Summer Tomato Soup 84
Sunday Beef Fathead 198
Superfood & Low-Protein Soup 118
Sweet Pork Chops with Brie Cheese 162
Sweet Pork Chops with Hoisin Sauce 171
Swiss Pork Patties with Salad 181

Taco Salad 67

V

W

Walnut Beef Skillet with Brussel Sprouts 203
Warm Cauliflower Salad 71
Warm Mushroom & Pepper Salad 75
Wild Mushroom Soup 122
Winter Chicken with Vegetables 148

Y

Yellow Squash Duck Breast Stew 133
Yummy Spareribs in Béarnaise Sauce 158

Z

Zesty Zucchini Bread with Nuts 7
Zucchini & Bell Pepper Chicken Gratin 141
Zucchini & Leek Turkey Soup 93
Zucchini & Pepper Caprese Gratin 21
Zucchini & Tomato Pork Omelet 156
Zucchini Casserole 44
Zucchini Soup 105
Zucchini Spread 36
Zuppa Toscana with Kale 85

Made in the USA
Middletown, DE
25 June 2023

33624651R00121